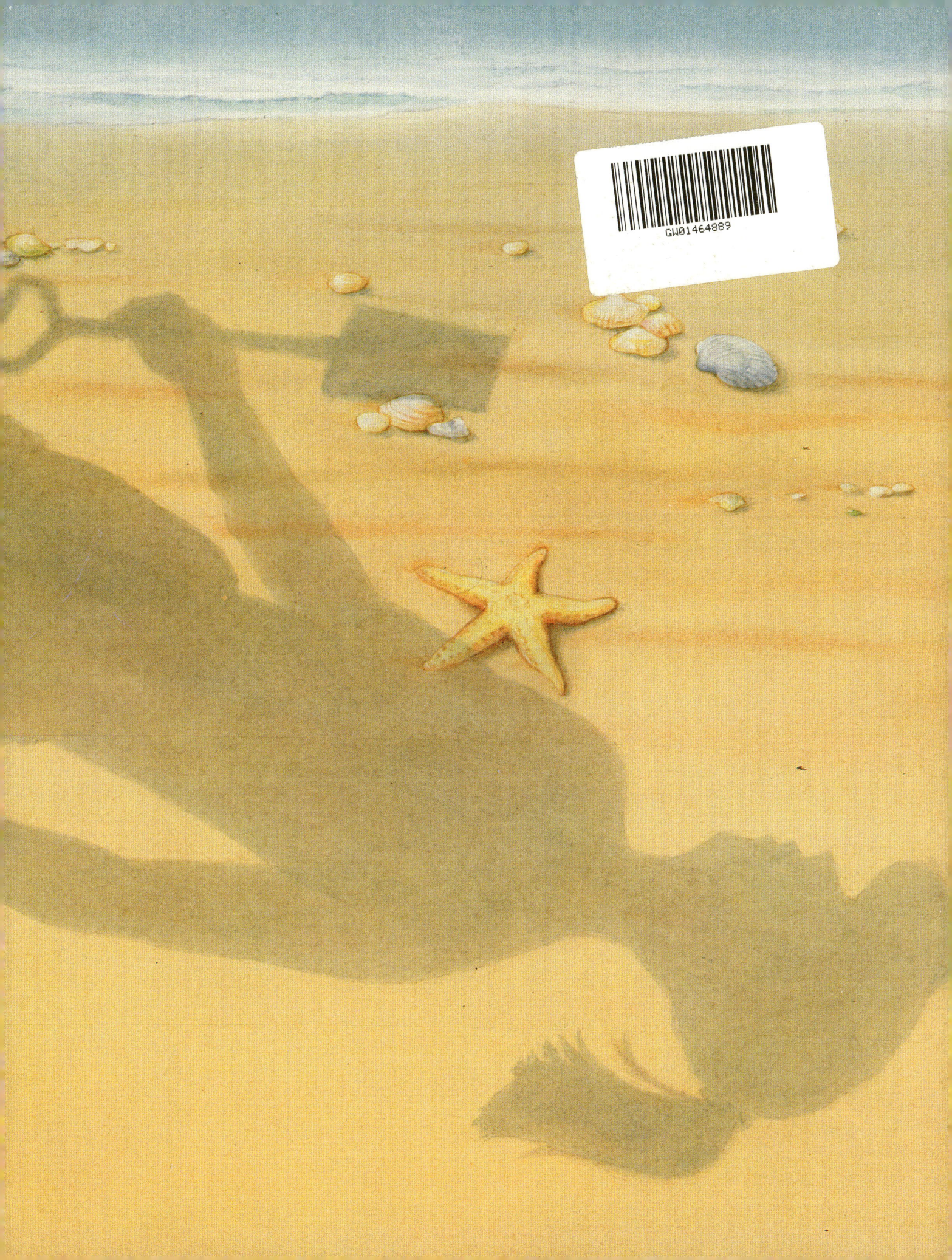

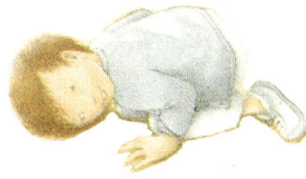

WRITTEN BY
CHANTAL HENRY-BIABAUD AND DORINE BARBEY,
MARTINE BECK, ROGER DIEVART

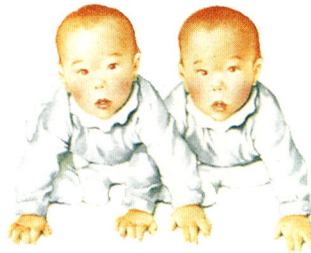

ILLUSTRATED BY
DANIEL BALAGE, LILIANE BLONDEL, DANIELE BOUR,
JEAN-PHILIPPE DUPONQ, JACQUES ROZIER AND MONIQUE GAUDRIAULT,
DONALD GRANT, FLORENCE HELMBACHER, GILBERT HOUBRE,
NATHALIE LOCOSTE, AGNES MATHIEU, CLAUDE AND DENISE MILLET,
SYLVAINE PEROLS, JEAN-MARIE POISSENOT, ALINE RIQUIER,
PIERRE-MARIE VALAT, DIZ WALLIS

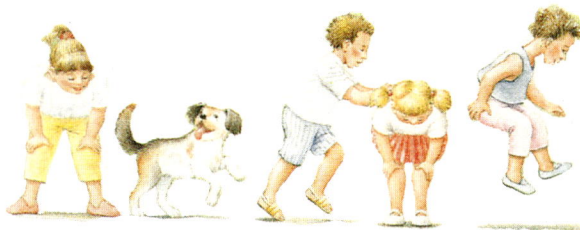

TRANSLATED AND ADAPTED BY
SARAH GIBSON
WITH SARAH MATTHEWS

We gratefully acknowledge the advice of:
Dr Andrew Gibson, M.B., B.Chir.
Gill Mather, Dental Health Adviser,
West Berkshire Health Authority
Geraldine Reid, D.Th.D., Nutritional and Dietary Therapist

Cover design by Peter Bennett
ISBN 1 85103 175 8
© 1991 by Editions Gallimard
English text © 1993
by Moonlight Publishing Ltd
First published in Great Britain 1993 by Moonlight Publishing Ltd,
36 Stratford Road, London W8
Printed in Italy by Editoriale Libraria

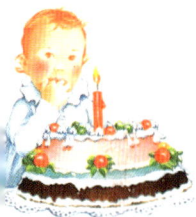

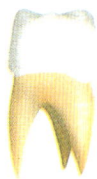

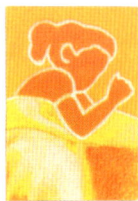

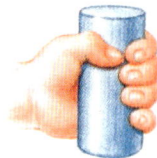

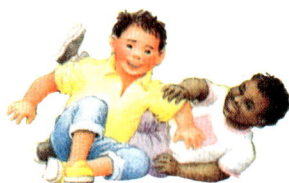

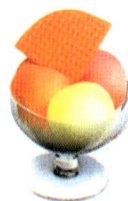

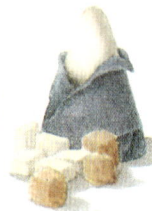

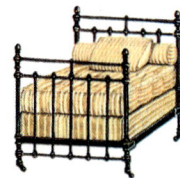

OUR BODY

CONTENTS

MOONLIGHT PUBLISHING

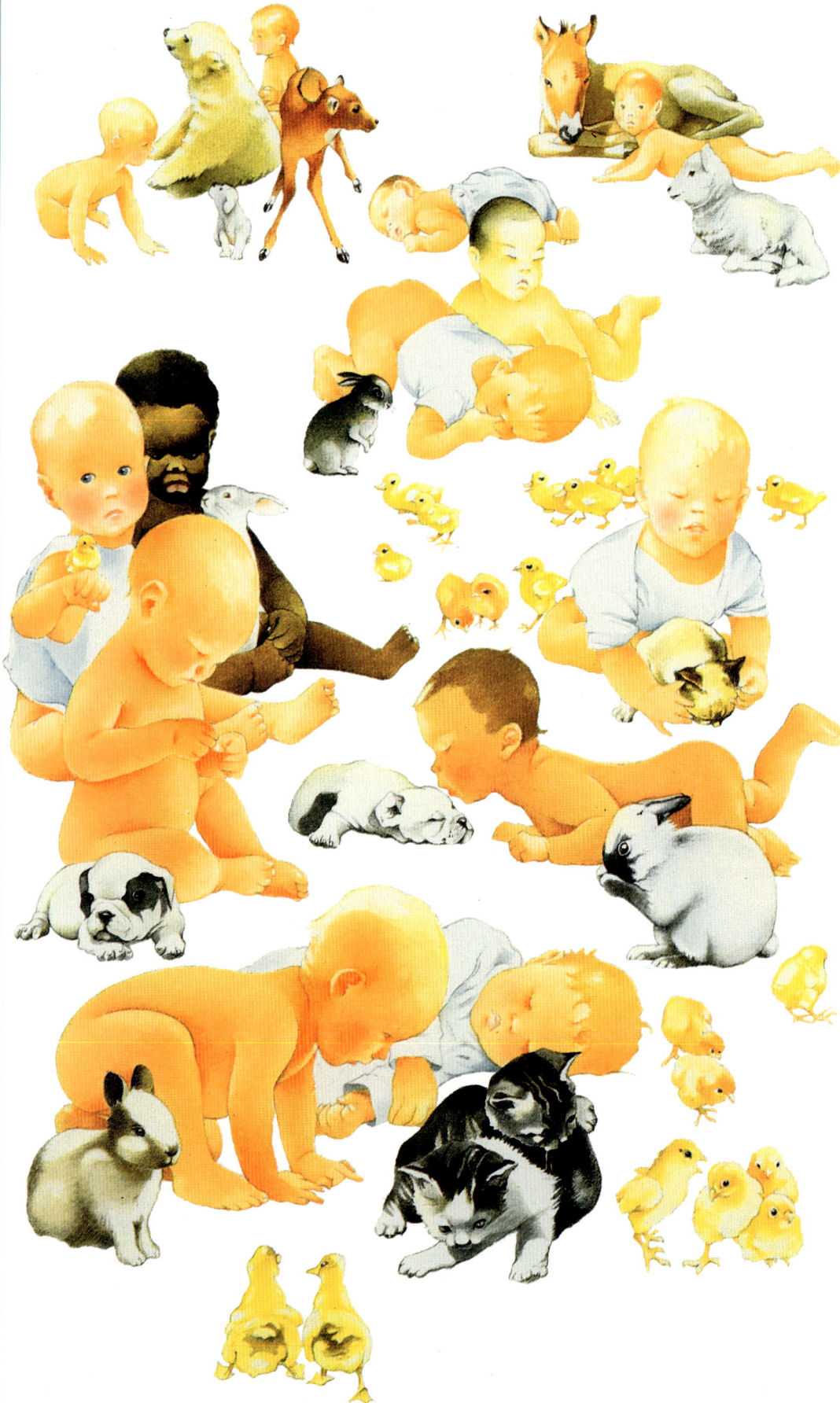

Short or tall; heavy or light; young or old; blond, red-headed, brown or black; fair, olive or dark skinned; the basic model is the same.

We each have a head with hair, two eyes, two ears, a nose, a mouth, a body with two arms and two legs, and we're each supported by a spine to keep us upright. It's not just coincidence that we are all made this way. It's because we all belong to the same species: you and I are human beings.

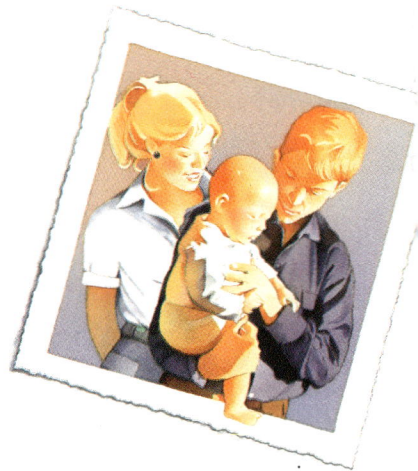

The human species is part of the larger animal kingdom. We are distinguished from other animals by our large and highly-developed brains, our use of language and our upright posture.

Babies come from their mothers' tummies.

Your birthday is your own special day, because it is the date when you were born.
All human babies come out of their mothers' tummies at birth. Although they are born in the same way, every one is different and special.

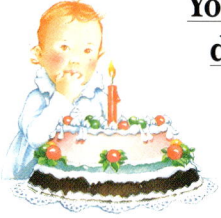

There are 250 babies being born somewhere in the world at every minute of the day and night. Each baby has a father and a mother: the parents were born from their mothers' tummies, too. Every animal has a father and a mother as well.

Not all animals are born in the same way.
Some hatch out of an egg laid by the mother. The egg has a store of food, so that the baby can grow, protected inside its shell. All birds lay eggs, and so do fish, insects and most reptiles. Tortoise and turtle eggs are round, not oval, with soft shells.

Once the mother tortoise has laid her eggs, she goes away and doesn't look after them. A baby tortoise has just hatched.

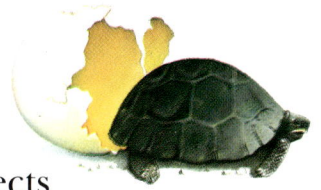

Ladybirds and other insects lay lots and lots of tiny, fragile eggs. They have to lay so many because only a few survive until they hatch.

A mother ladybird lays her eggs after the father has fertilized* them.

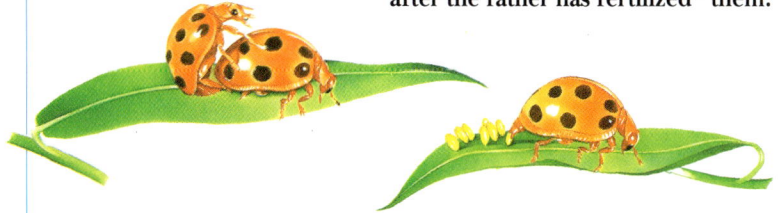

All baby mammals grow inside the mother, just as human babies do.
Have you ever seen puppies or kittens drinking milk from their mother? All animals that spend their early days suckling milk from their mothers are called mammals.
You are a mammal, too.

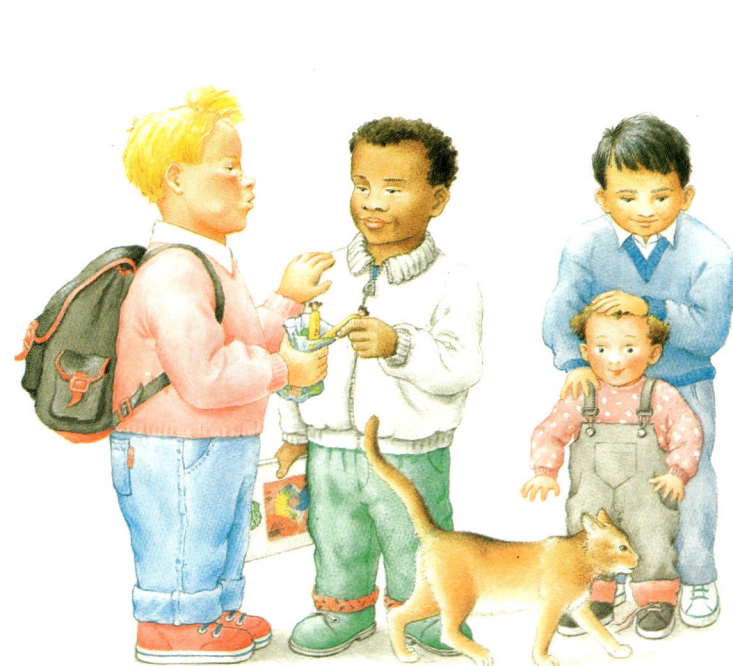

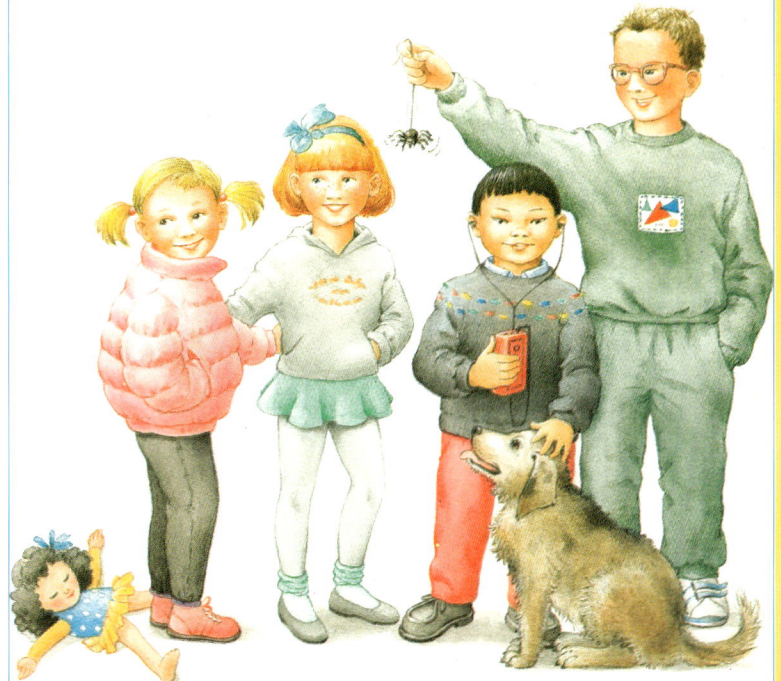

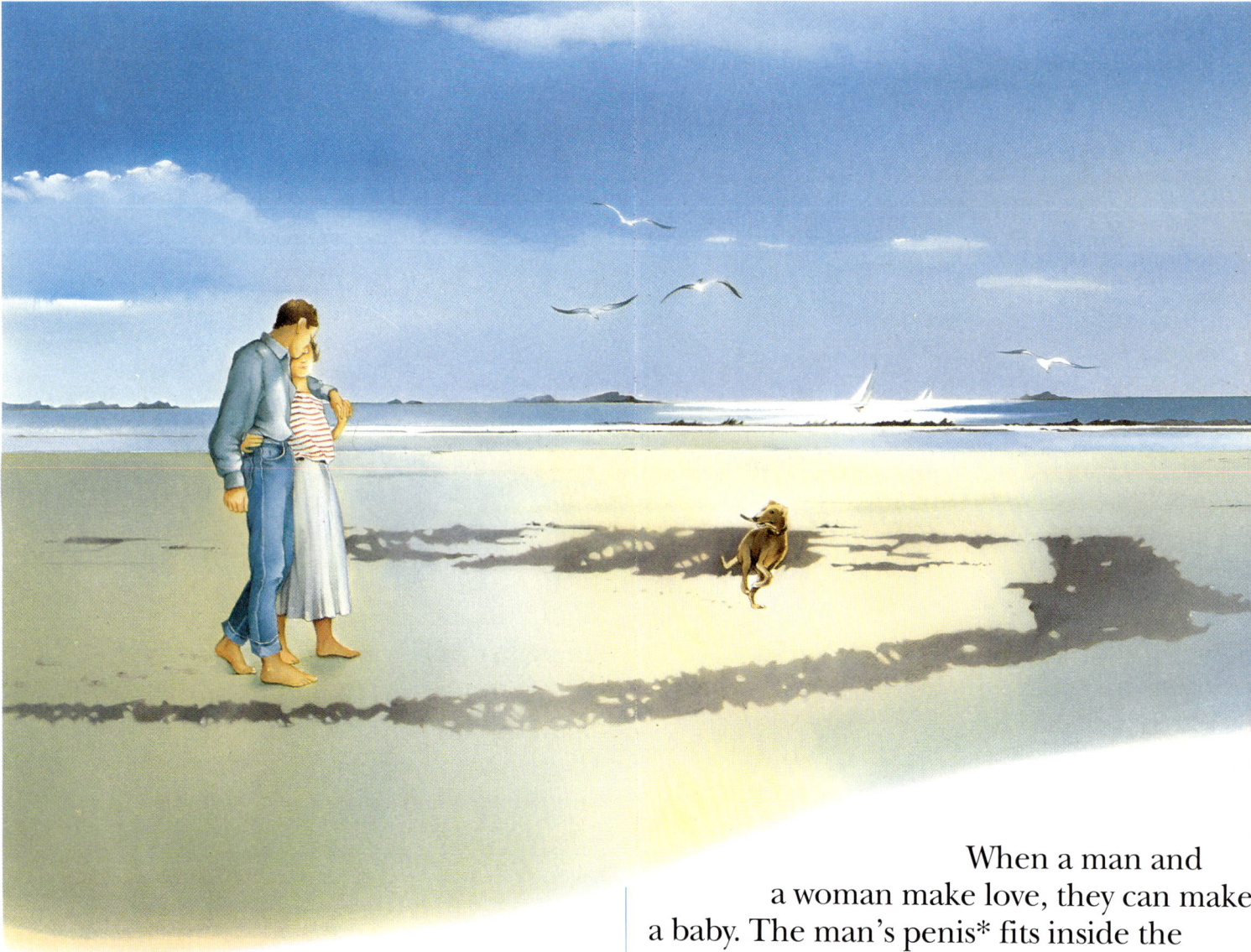

When a man and a woman love each other, they enjoy being together, holding each other, walking and talking, making plans for the future. They want to live together and share their love by having children.

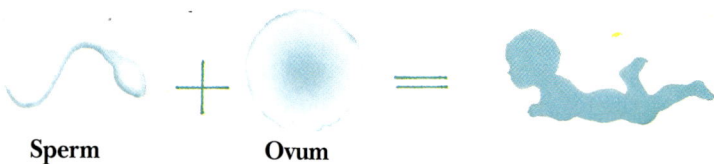

Sperm + Ovum =

Sperm   **Ovum**

A man and a woman each have inside them half of what is needed to make a baby: a man has the sperm and a woman has the egg cell, the ovum.

When a man and a woman make love, they can make a baby. The man's penis* fits inside the woman's vagina* and releases a liquid full of sperms. There may be millions of sperms, but only one of them will manage to penetrate the woman's ovum.

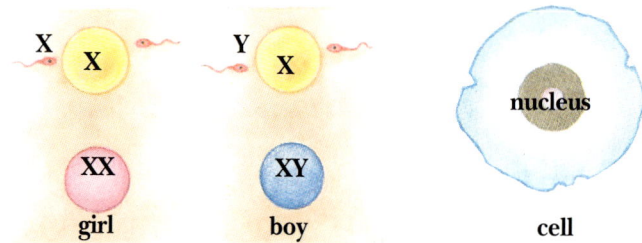

X X   Y X

XX   XY

girl   **boy**

nucleus

cell

Fertilization: the sperm and ovum meet.
One sperm and one ovum join together to form an egg, this one cell will grow into a new baby.

You started as one tiny cell, unlike any other.

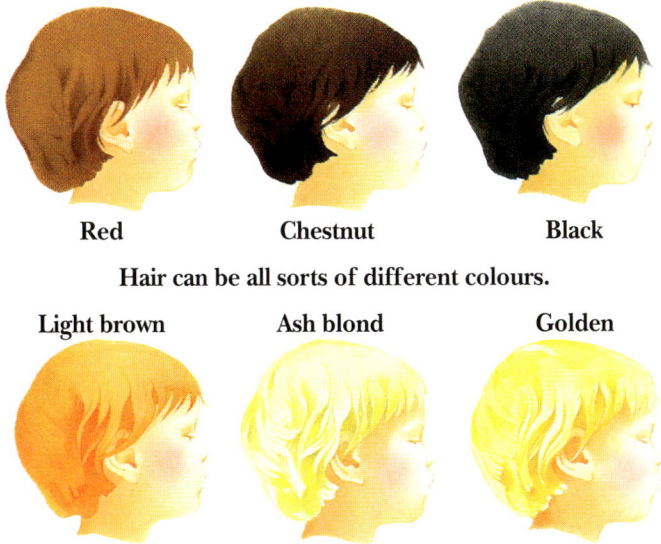

Red   Chestnut   Black

Hair can be all sorts of different colours.

Light brown   Ash blond   Golden

All the characteristics of the new baby are there in the nucleus* of the first cell.

They are written on tiny thread-like chromosomes, which are made up of thousands of genes*. They carry in their memory all the information passed on by the parents. There are genes for everything: the colour of the baby's skin, its eyes and its hair, how tall it will grow, the shape of its ears. That's why you might have blue eyes like your mother, or a turned-up nose like your father.

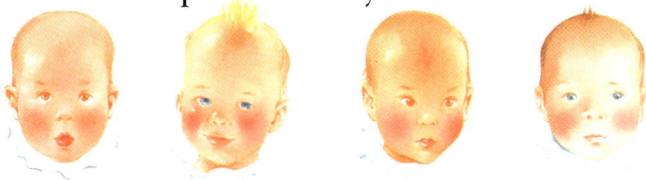

Will the baby be a girl or a boy?

It depends which sperm reaches the ovum. Inside the ovum, the chromosome which decides the baby's sex is always in the shape of an X. In the sperm, it is sometimes X-shaped, and sometimes Y-shaped. If a sperm with an X chromosome joins the ovum, they will produce an XX cell and the baby will be a girl. If the ovum meets a Y chromosome, they will produce an XY cell and the baby will be a boy.

What about twins?

Sometimes, the mother produces two ova. If two sperms manage to fertilize the two eggs, two babies will start to develop at the same time. They won't be identical twins: one might be a boy, the other a girl.

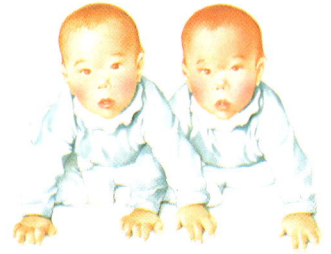

Occasionally, the fertilized ovum divides into two, and the two parts go on to form identical twins. They are always the same sex and they look very like each other. A mother can have three, four, five or even six babies at the same time... but that is very unusual!
The egg takes nine months to develop in the uterus, a very supple muscle in the mother's tummy which stretches and gets bigger as the baby inside grows.

These nine months are called pregnancy.

Inside the uterus the baby lies cradled in a bag of watery fluid, which protects it from bumps as its mother gets on with daily life. The umbilical cord links the baby to the placenta, which is rather like a sponge fastened to the wall of the uterus.

At one month, the egg is the size of a pea.
At this stage, we call it an embryo.
The heart begins to beat at six weeks old.

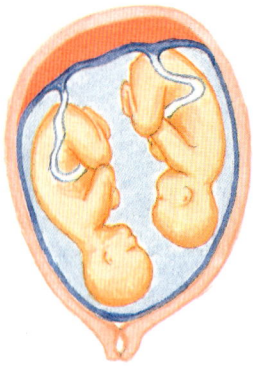

Identical twins grow in the same bag of fluid and share the same placenta.

How does the mother feed her baby while it's in her tummy?

Blood passes through the placenta and along the umbilical cord, carrying nutrients, water and oxygen to the baby, and taking waste matter away. A woman who is expecting a baby gets tired easily, even before her tummy begins to get bigger.

How does the embryo grow inside its mother?

At two months, the embryo has grown to the size of a walnut. Its head and its limbs are starting to appear, like buds. It has the beginnings of fingers and toes. There are already outlines where its ears will be, and its eyes are covered with eyelids.

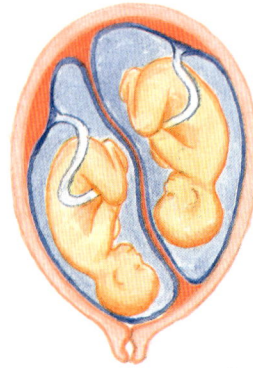

Non-identical twins grow in separate bags, and each has its own placenta.

At three months,

the embryo is beginning to look like a miniature baby. It is now called the foetus (pronounced 'feetus'). It is 7 centimetres long, and is starting to swallow and make its first movements.

At four months,

the foetus sleeps a lot during the day, when its mother is moving around. Then in the evening, when she relaxes, it begins to move its head, its arms and legs.

At five months,

the mother can feel the baby moving. It kicks and turns somersaults, trying to find the most comfortable position. Its hair begins to grow. It can swallow the fluid that surrounds it, and suck its thumb.

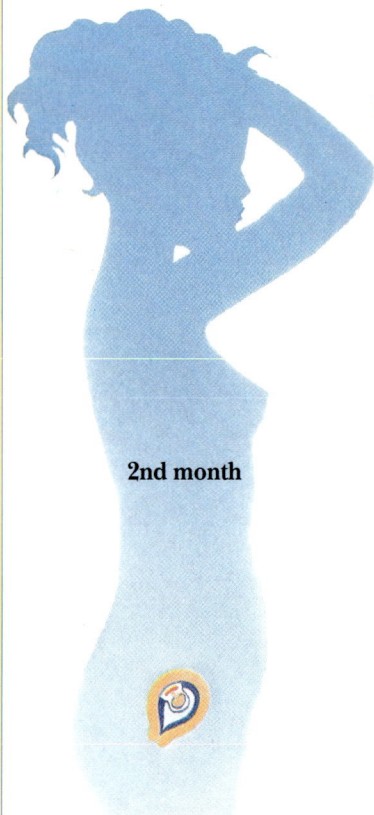

2nd month

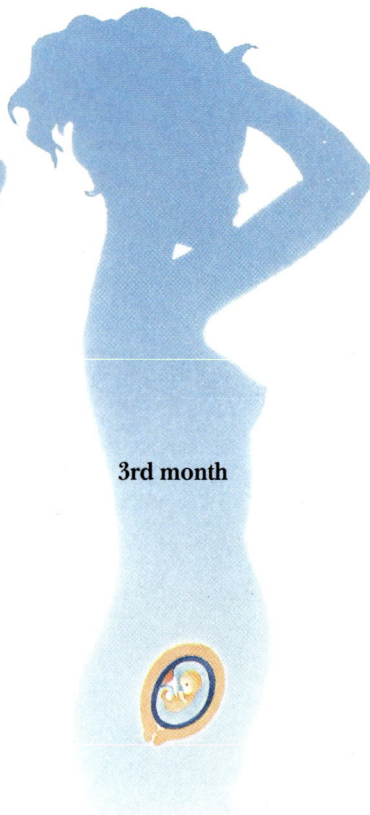

3rd month

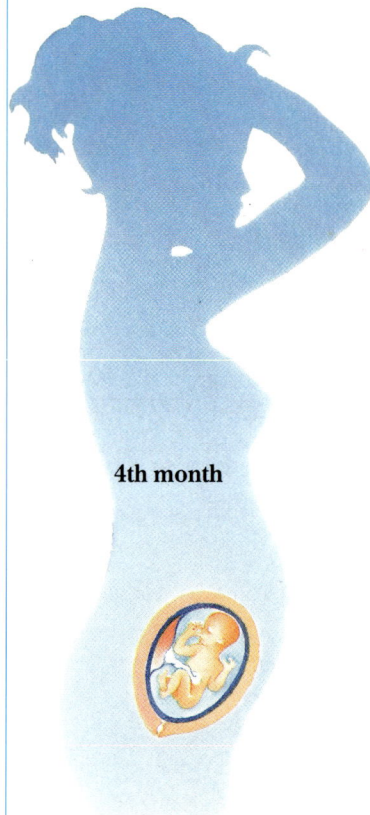

4th month

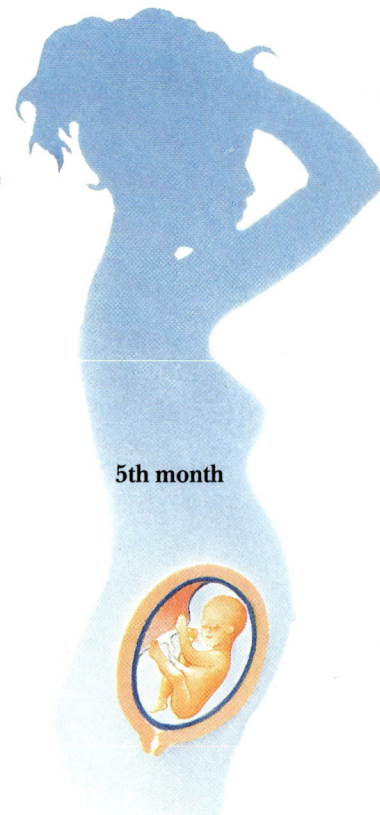

5th month

At six months,

the foetus weighs one kilo.
When it has drunk too much, it gets
hiccups which makes its mother's tummy
jump! It can pee, and has finger nails.
Its skin, which was so fine and delicate,
is now growing stronger. It's getting fatter,
curling into a ball, because there doesn't
seem to be so much space anymore! It can
hear sounds, muffled by the fluid around
it, but a piercing cry can make it jump.

At seven months,

it opens its eyes. It enjoys hearing sounds
made by its mother's body, the beating
of her heart, the sound of her voice.
It's moving a lot now, kicking and
punching because there's not much
room left.

The foetus (1), the placenta (2) and the bag of amniotic fluid (3) inside the uterus (4). Umbilical cord (5)

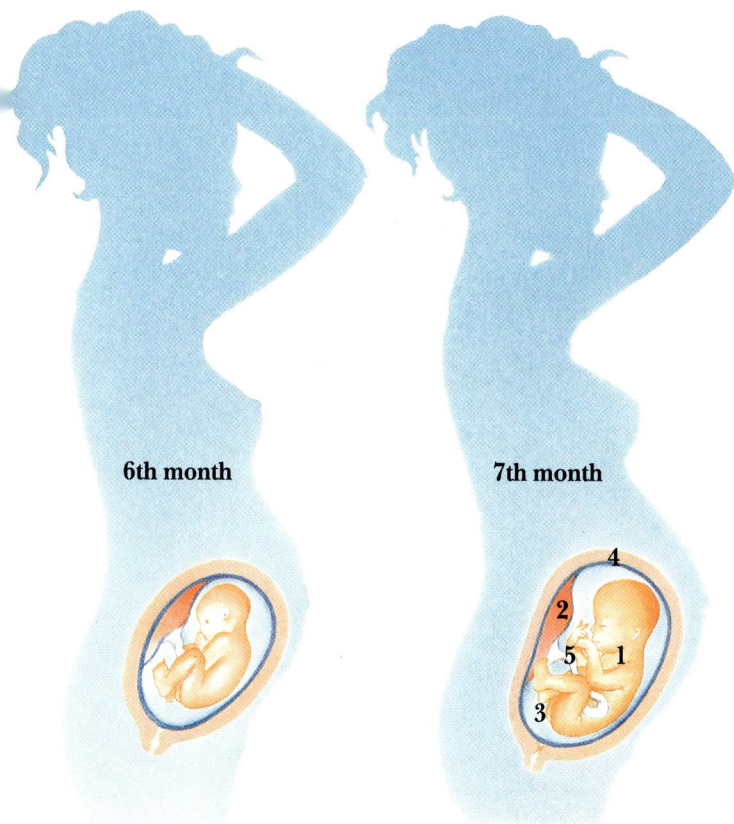

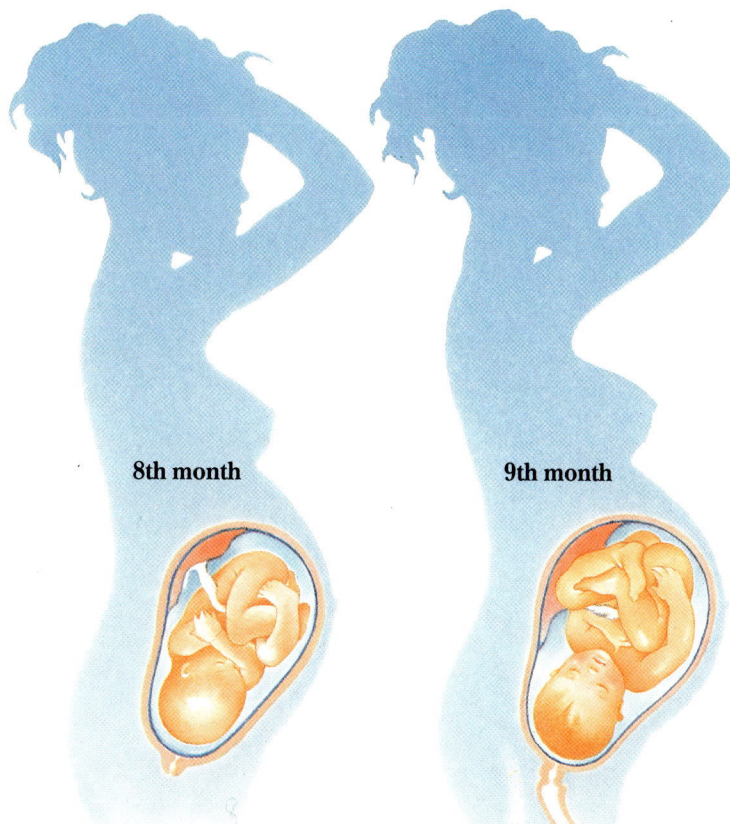

At eight months,

it has grown so big that it can't turn
somersaults inside its mother any more!
Its tiny tongue is already able to taste.
Everything is finished: all it needs is to put
on a little more weight. Its head is usually
pointing downwards, ready to be born.

At nine months,

it weighs about three kilos.
The baby is usually born after nine months
in the uterus, but sometimes it is born
earlier. A baby that is born before the eighth
month is called a premature baby. It has
not had time to finish growing, and it is very
weak and delicate. Its lungs are not fully
developed. Premature babies are put into
incubators, little heated cots where they
can be looked after carefully.

6th month

7th month

8th month

9th month

The time comes for the baby to be born.

The mother knows when she is going to give birth. She starts to get pains in her tummy, as her muscles contract to push the baby towards the opening of the uterus. We call this 'labour', because birth is hard work for mother and baby!

At last the baby comes out through the mother's vagina, which stretches to allow the baby to be born. Usually, the head appears first, followed by the rest of the body. The placenta, or afterbirth, follows about twenty minutes later.

Babies have a little soft space between the bones of their skulls: the fontanelle.

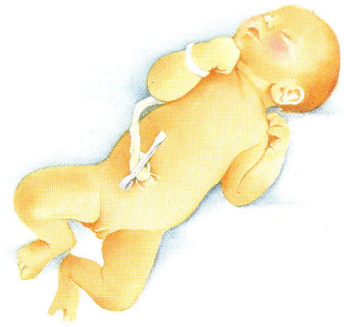

Soon her umbilical cord will drop off.

Birth must be quite a shock for the baby!

For nine months, it's been in the dark in a warm liquid, and suddenly there is light and noise. It begins to cry, a sign that it is breathing well. The umbilical cord is no longer needed: it can be cut without hurting mother or child. When held up, a new-born baby can move its legs as if trying to walk. If a baby is born in hospital, a bracelet with its name on is strapped on its wrist, so that nobody can get mixed up!

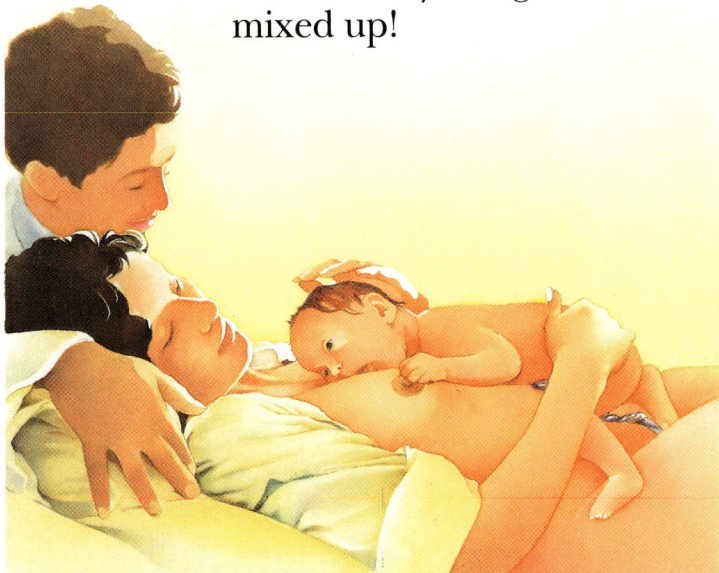

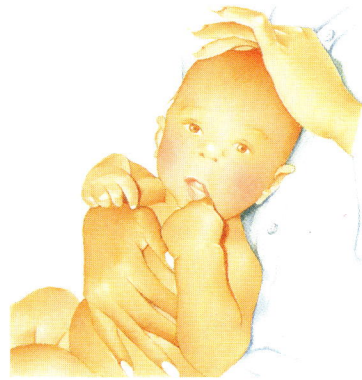

A new-born baby may be very tiny, but it is very important to its parents from the moment it is born. One of the first things that they do is to give their child a name.

Do you have one first name, or several?

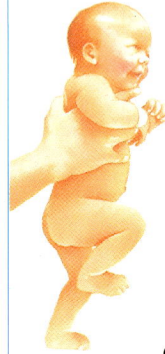

Do you know why your parents chose your names? Customs vary, depending on the nationality and culture you belong to. In Thailand, every baby is called Nou, meaning 'little mouse', until it is one month old. Then a name is chosen for it according to the day on which it was born. In Kashmir, children are only given their own names when they are four or five years old.

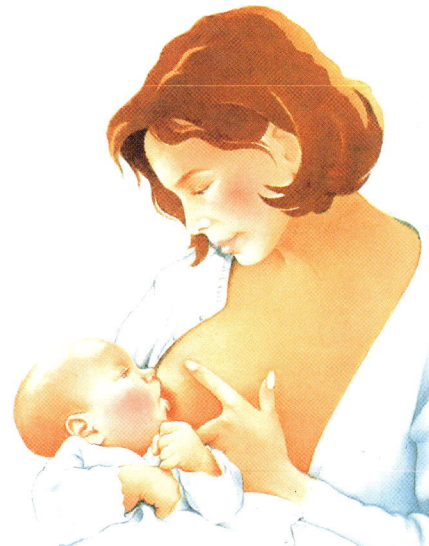

As soon as a baby is born, it is able to suck milk from its mother's nipple.

A baby's first days

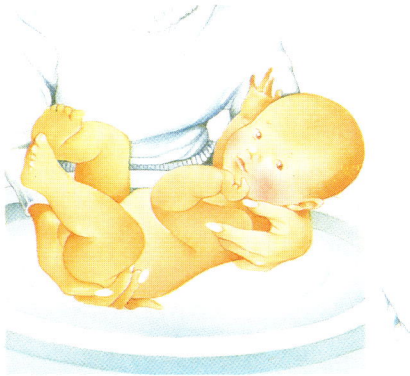
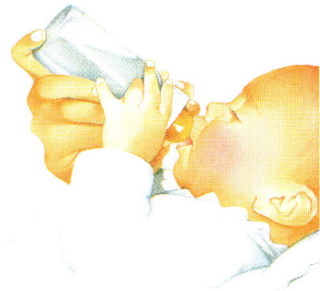

Babies love having baths...   ...and being fed.

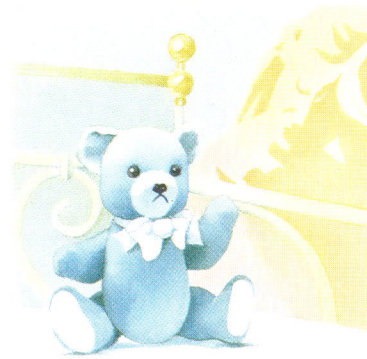
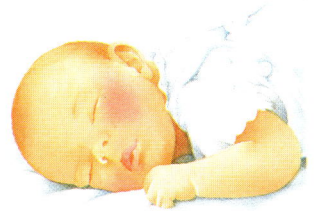

Babies see best what is close. They sleep a lot of the time.

Babies are often hungry.
Before the baby was born, she was fed all the time, day and night, through the umbilical cord. Now, she lets her mother know she is hungry by crying. For the first weeks, she feeds every three to four hours, drinking milk from her mother's breast or from a bottle. Gradually, she is given something other than milk, and can go slightly longer between feeds.

A baby loves to be cuddled by her parents, or by an older brother or sister. She likes the warm feeling and smell of people who love her, and whom she knows best. She is learning about the outside world through contact with them. Loud noises and sudden movements are frightening.

After a few days, the remains of the baby's umbilical cord drop off, leaving a small scar: the tummy button.
Babies can't see very well at first.
They only see shapes and bright colours.

It is important that a baby puts on weight.
At first, she is weighed at least once a week to make sure she is growing properly.
She puts on about 30 grams a day for the first two months.
After a while, she is weighed every month or so. A baby should put on weight quite quickly. If she is not gaining weight, or even is losing weight, it may be a sign that all is not well.

Mothers the world over choose
different ways of carrying their babies.

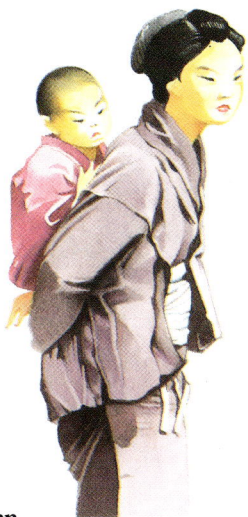
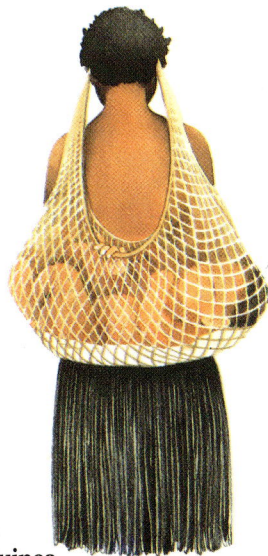
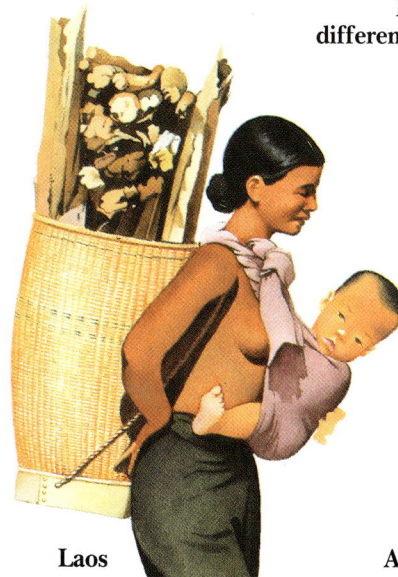
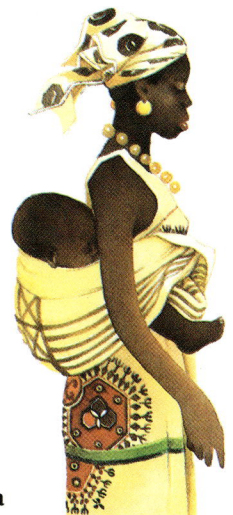

Japan

Papua-
New Guinea

Laos

Africa

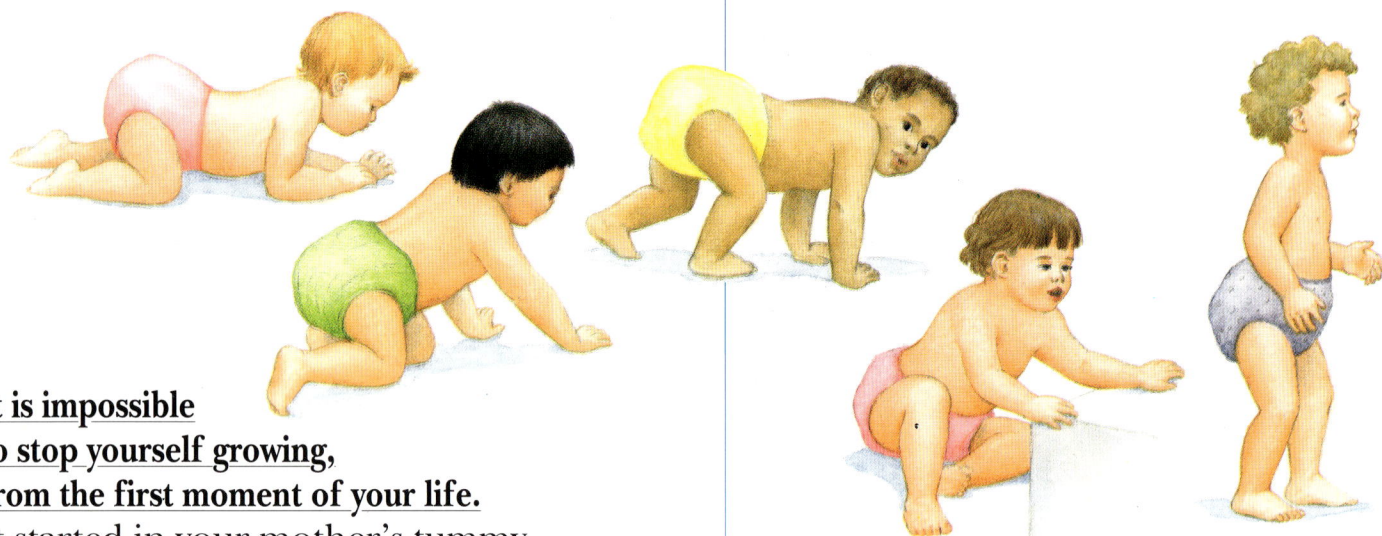

**It is impossible
to stop yourself growing,
from the first moment of your life.**
It started in your mother's tummy,
when you were still an embryo and then
a foetus. The new-born baby grows bigger,
turns into a child, then an adolescent
and finally an adult.
When you are young, you grow very fast.
Those shoes that were bought just a couple
of months ago are already tight. And last
winter's trousers are much too small now!
Ever since the first cell divided, long
before you were born, the cells of your
body have been multiplying, forming
different tissues*.

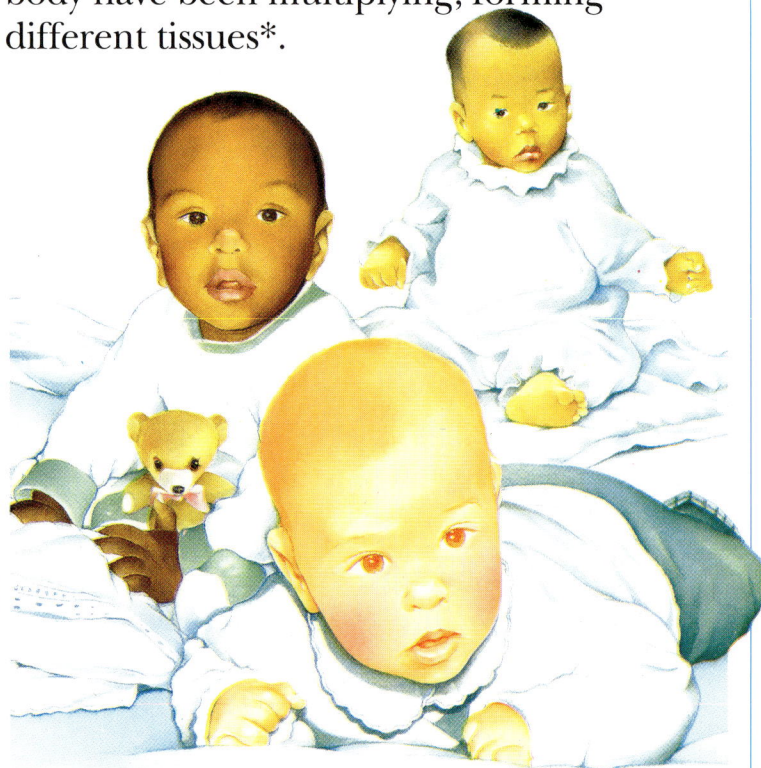

The tissues of your body are grouped
together to make up its different organs.
Cells are the building blocks of your body.
The genes in your chromosomes dictate
what you will be like as you grow up.
Half are passed on from one parent, half
from the other, which explains why you
may be tall like your father, or why you
may have more of your mother's build.
Your cells are changing all the time: those
that are too old are replaced by new ones.
In the first weeks of life, you simply grow
in weight and length. Then you start to
learn different things: your senses develop
and your bones get harder and stronger.
Every organ, every part of your body has
a timetable of growth. There may be times
when your feet seem too big for the rest
of you, or your mouth seems crowded
with teeth that are too large. Don't worry:
this is quite normal. Your body will sort
itself out in the end.

A final big change: adolescence
During these few years, the boy becomes
a man, and the girl becomes a woman.
They are now adults, capable of having
children of their own.

Hormones are the body's chemical messengers.
They are released into the blood from
little glands. Hormones from the pituitary*
gland control growth: they are especially
hard at work during puberty.
Puberty is the time during the growing-up
process when the parts of the body that
are there for making babies begin to work.
This happens during pre-adolescence and
adolescence, between the age of ten
and sixteen for girls, and around twelve
to fourteen for boys.

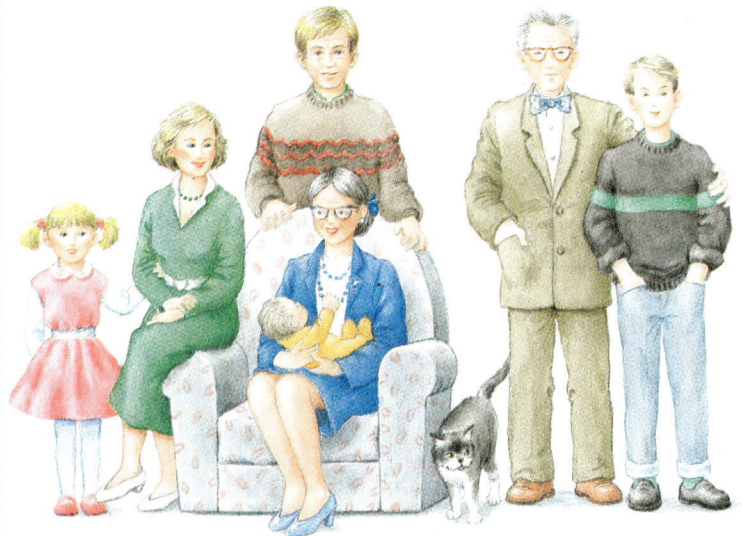

Our personalities grow stronger as we
become more independent, but it isn't
always easy to feel comfortable in a body
which is changing so fast. Sometimes your
mood swings up and down, and as for
parents – they can be so frustrating!
Be patient: they love you, but they've
got to adjust to the changes in you too!

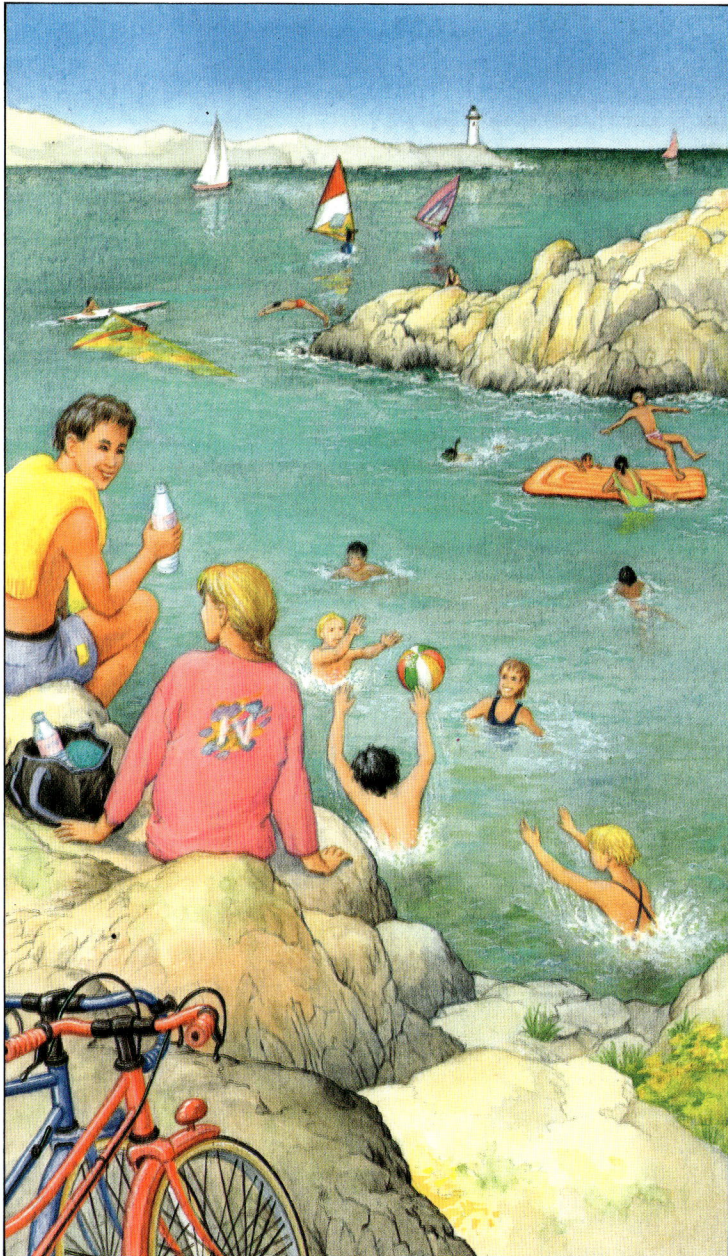

**A balanced diet and plenty of vitamins are vital
for a strong, healthy body.**
The unseen things are important, too:
the love and attention of your family, friends
and school will help build self-esteem and
a healthy personality.

Grown-ups have finished growing.
Between the ages of 20 and 30, the body
is at its strongest and the brain at its most
alert. As we get older, our cells renew
themselves more slowly, so it takes longer
to repair damaged or diseased parts of
the body. Finally, like the worn-out engine
of an old car, our heart stops and we die.
But life goes on, as children grow up, get
married and have babies in their turn.

Food goes on a long journey through the digestive system.

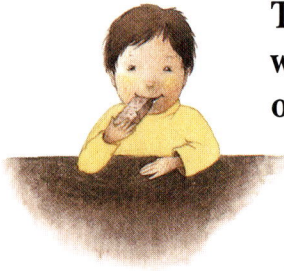

To help your body live, work well and do any repairs, it is organized into different systems which divide up the work. The system that deals with food and waste is called the digestive system.

The food and drink we swallow has to be broken down into tiny particles by our digestive system before it can pass into the blood stream and give us the energy we need to live.

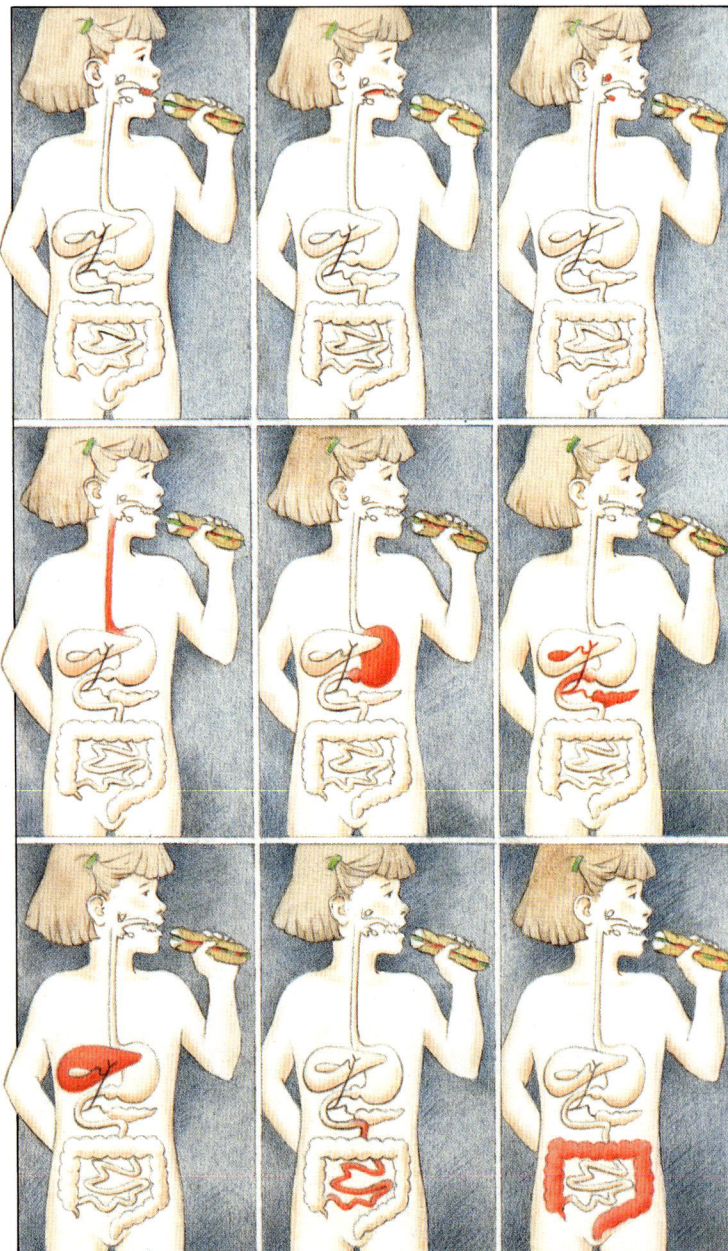

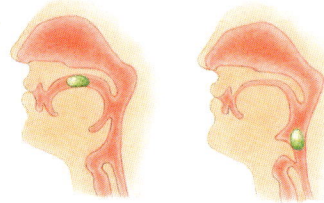

When you swallow, the epiglottis shuts off the opening to your windpipe like a lid, so that food doesn't go down into your lungs.

Your digestive system is like a very long tube which begins at your mouth and ends at your anus. In an adult, it's about 9 metres long, most of it coiled up in the abdomen!

How does the digestive system work?

Digestion starts with a mouthful of food which is chewed and mixed with saliva* until it is soft and mushy. Then you swallow, and the food goes down the oesophagus to your stomach. There it is mixed with digestive juices which are acid and dilute the food into a thick, soupy liquid. Muscles squeeze it along a little at a time into the small intestine, where useful particles of food called nutrients are separated from the undigestible waste. Nutrients pass into the bloodstream across the lining of the small intestine on their way to feed the body's cells. Undigested waste continues on through the large intestine and leaves your body through the anus as faeces when you go to the toilet.

Oesophagus

Liver

Stomach

Small intestine

Large intestine

Appendix

Anus

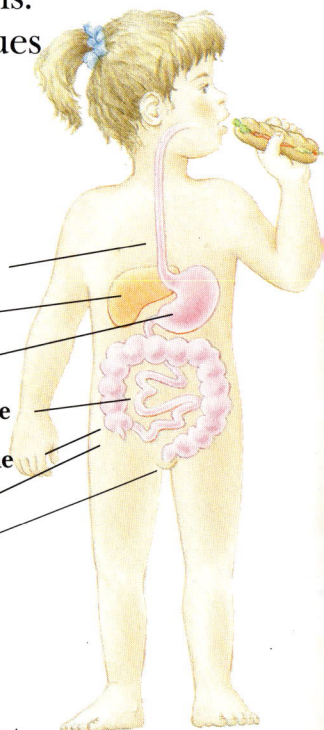

Digestive system seen from the front

Most of the nutrients that have passed into the bloodstream go to the liver before travelling to the rest of the body. The liver works like a factory, processing nutrients to feed the cells and storing vitamins. Blood is cleaned by our kidneys, which turn any waste into urine.

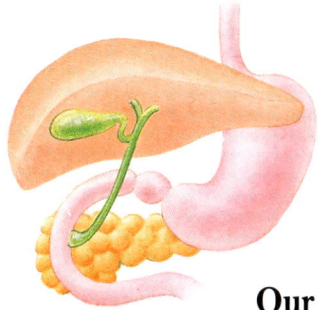

A liquid called bile pours from the liver into the small intestine to help digest fats.

Our digestive system is very complicated, so there is more than one reason why we sometimes get a stomach ache.
If you have eaten too much, you may feel sick. That's a form of indigestion. If you have swallowed germs, or eaten something that isn't fresh, you may get food poisoning. Your stomach won't accept the food, instead it contracts strongly and sends the food gushing back upwards, making you sick. If your intestine reacts as well, contracting rapidly to get rid of the bad food, you have diarrhoea.

Someone with 'heartburn' is in fact having trouble with their stomach. They've probably got indigestion.

A virus can make you ill with gastro-enteritis*. You may also get a tummy ache if you are nervous or annoyed. If you don't eat enough fibre and drink enough water, you may become constipated*, which can be painful. Wholemeal bread, prunes or high-fibre cereal, and plenty of water should put things right again.

Appendicitis
If the tiny appendix at the bottom of your large intestine becomes infected, it can give you a bad pain in your tummy. It has to be taken out with a little operation.

Unwanted visitors
Occasionally, you might get worms in your tummy. Some are tiny, others larger. A special medicine will quickly get rid of them! If you've had them, you must keep your nails short, because the worms' eggs can lodge underneath when you scratch yourself, and then you might pass them on to the rest of the family.

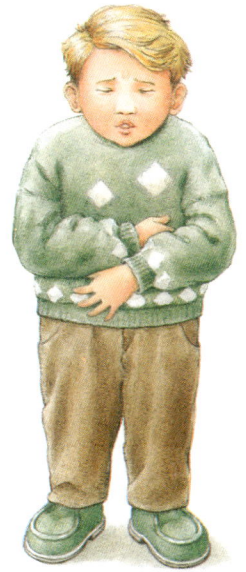

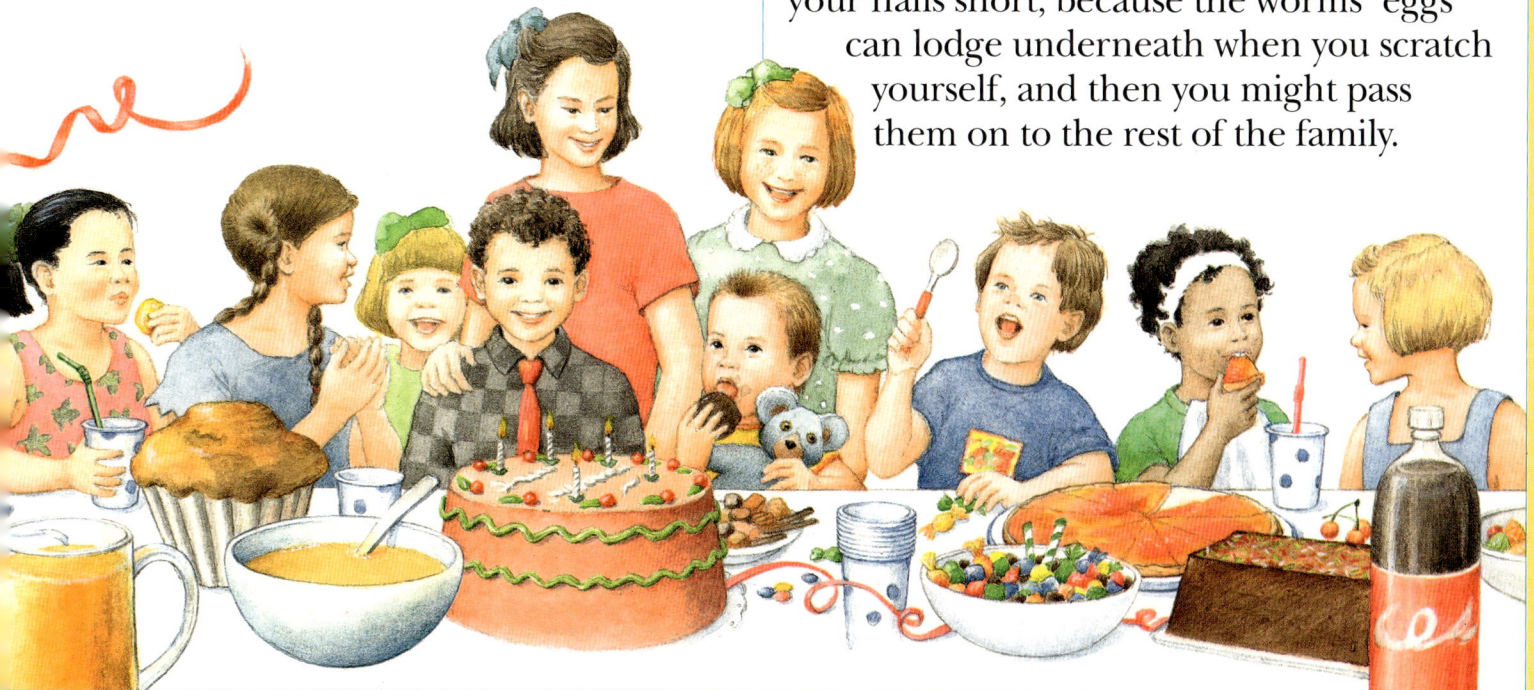

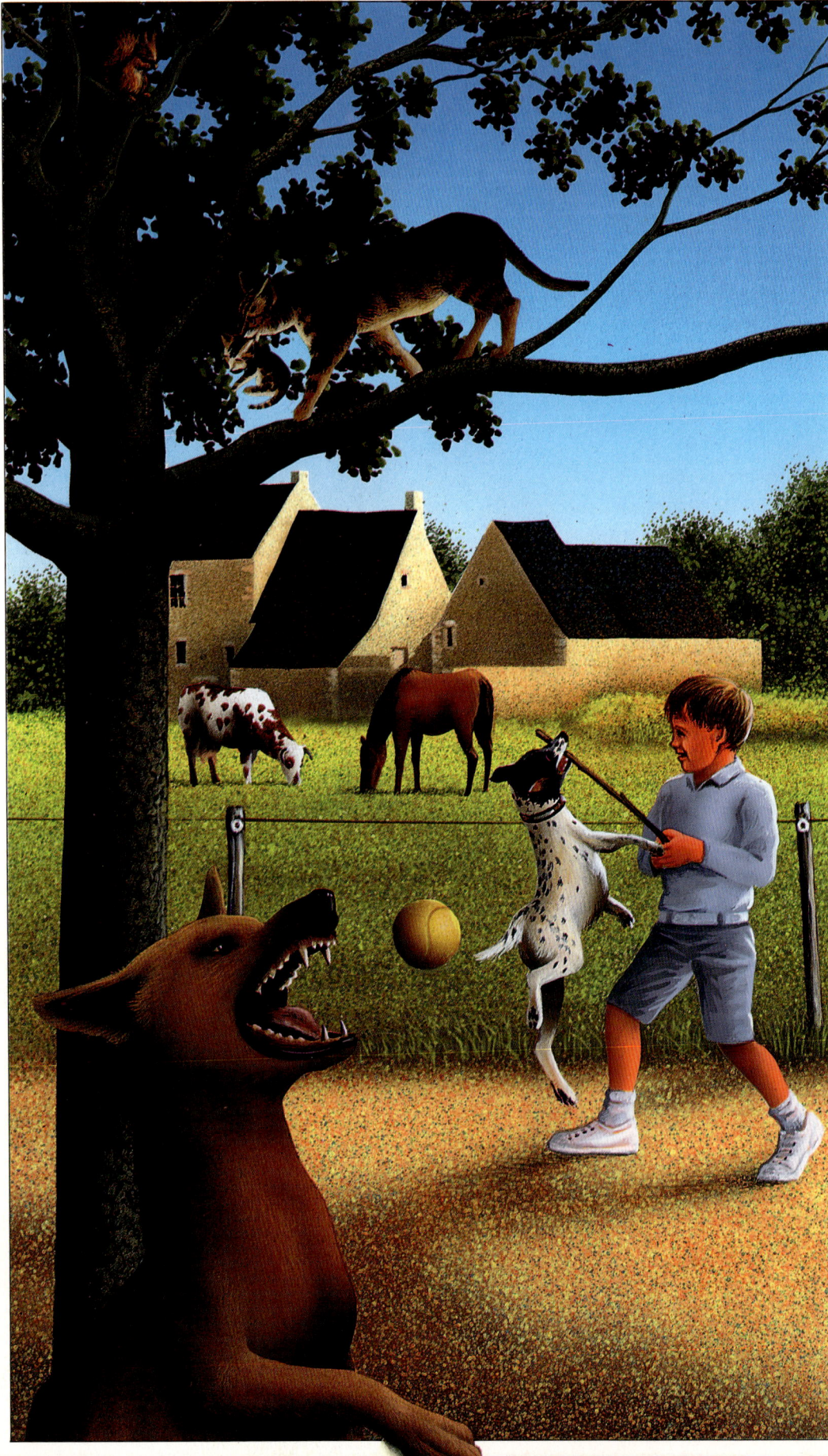

Teeth look nice, and they're very useful. They bite, chew, nibble, munch, crunch, tear, grind, gnaw... Just try eating without them!

Animals use their teeth for lots of things – even for carrying their babies.

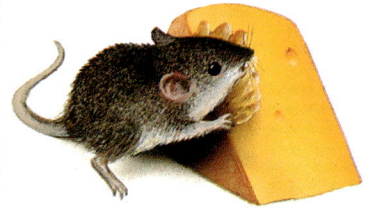

Teeth are different shapes and do different jobs.
The incisors at the front cut like a chisel. Next come the canine teeth – they're pointed, good for tearing up food. The big, flat teeth at the back are molars. You use them to chew your food.

Your mouth is like a cave.
The roof of your mouth is called the palate and at the far, dark end there's the uvula. Your tongue rolls your food around and sends it down your throat.

Teeth are little bones planted in your gums.

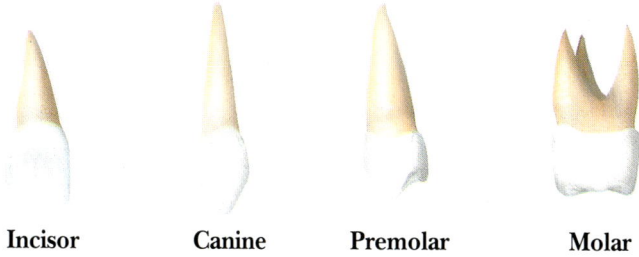

Incisor   Canine   Premolar   Molar

Teeth are living things.
They may not look like it, but they are in fact little bones.

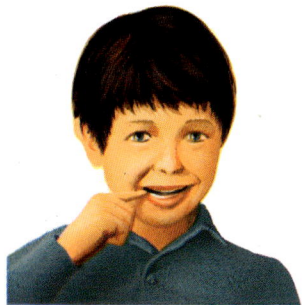

Teeth are fixed into the jawbones. The upper jaw does not move, the lower one can go up and down and from side to side.

What is a tooth made of?
What we see is the shiny white enamel (1), which is harder than bone. It protects your teeth from knocks, and from heat and cold, as well as from all the germs which live in your mouth.

Underneath, the dentine (2) protects the pulp (3), a soft tissue holding blood vessels (4) which feed the tooth and nerves (5). Have you ever had toothache? It's the nerves that make you feel the pain.

Just like a tree, with its roots in the soil, a tooth has its roots in the gum (6) and is firmly embedded in the jawbone. The part above the gum is called the crown. The part you can't see is called the root.

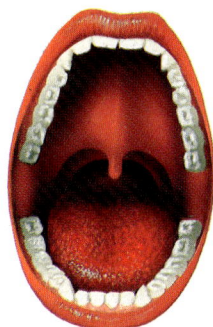

Mouth

You use the incisors at the front of your mouth when you bite into an apple.

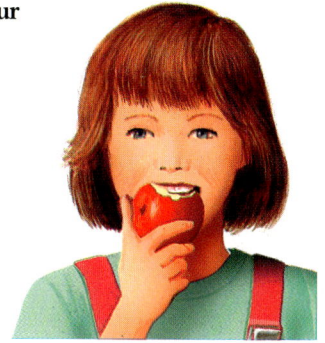

All these things are very good for your teeth:
water containing fluoride; fish, milk, butter, cheese, eggs... all contain calcium, a mineral which keeps your teeth strong. Fresh fruit and green vegetables contain vitamin C, to give you healthy gums.

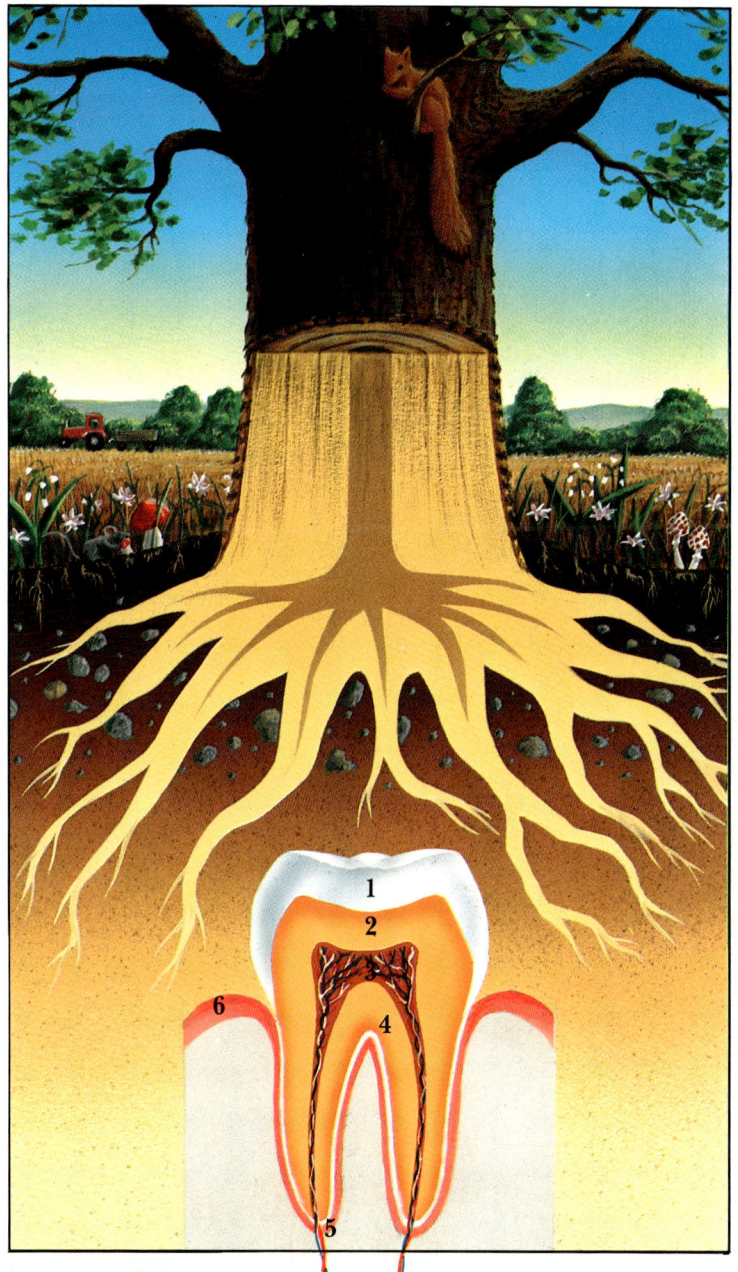

Milk teeth and permanent teeth

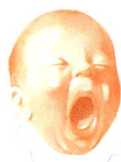

First teeth

Babies don't usually have any teeth when they are born. Apparently King Louis XIV of France was born with a tooth! But it's very rare.

When a baby is about six months old, its cheeks look red, it cries and dribbles a lot. Then a first tooth appears: a lower incisor. We say the baby is 'cutting teeth'. It hurts because the teeth are, literally, cutting through the gum. The poor baby is grumpy, and sometimes has a fever.

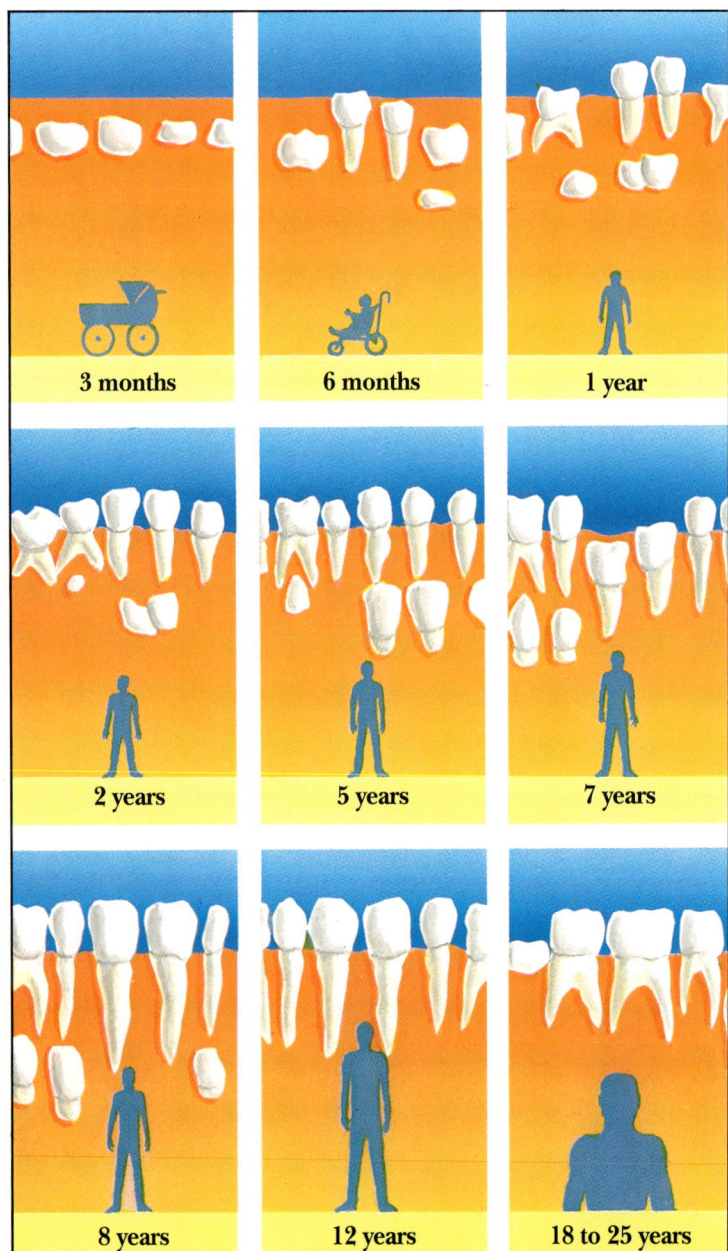

1. Incisors do the cutting and slicing.

2. Canines do the cutting and tearing.

3. Premolars grind and chew.

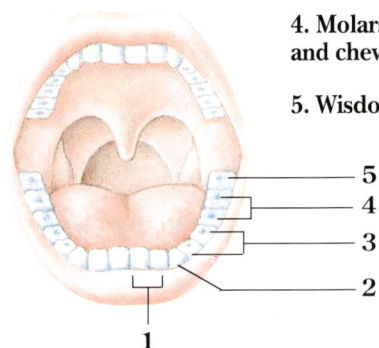

4. Molars grind and chew.

5. Wisdom teeth

The lower incisors are the first to appear, followed by the upper ones. Then come the canines, and then the molars.

At two and a half years old, a child has twenty teeth, called 'milk teeth' because they appear during the time the baby is drinking a lot of milk. Later, between the ages of six and eleven, these fall out, pushed out of the way by the second set of teeth. It hardly hurts at all.

Teeth for life

Underneath each milk tooth, there's another tooth waiting to grow and replace it.

X-rays show what your eyes can't see: under the milk teeth, the permanent teeth waiting to grow.

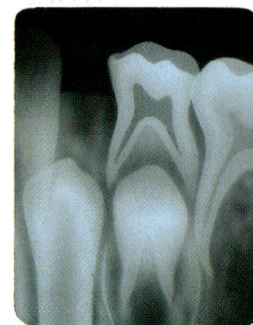

When you're about 18, the last teeth to appear come through. They are the large molars at the back, called wisdom teeth, because you're supposed to be wise by the time they grow... Some people never get them.

An adult has thirty-two teeth in all: eight incisors, four canines, eight premolars, twelve molars.

3 months	6 months	1 year
2 years	5 years	7 years
8 years	12 years	18 to 25 years

Take good care of your teeth!

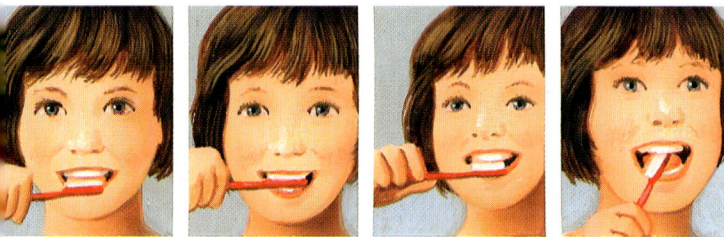

A long time ago, people used their teeth much more than we do today.

Their teeth were very strong. They were used to crunching raw vegetables, and could tear and bite raw meat. There were no sugary sweets to eat.

This is how a dentist fills a cavity.

What did you do if you had toothache in the olden days?

There were no dentists. You might try to help the pain with herbs, but if it got too bad, you could go to a travelling tooth-puller. He would yank the bad tooth out, while a musician played loudly to drown the yells!

How often should you go to the dentist?

At least once a year, to have a check-up. If your tooth is sensitive to cold or heat, go straightaway – you may have a small hole, or cavity. If infection gets into the pulp, it will hurt a lot.

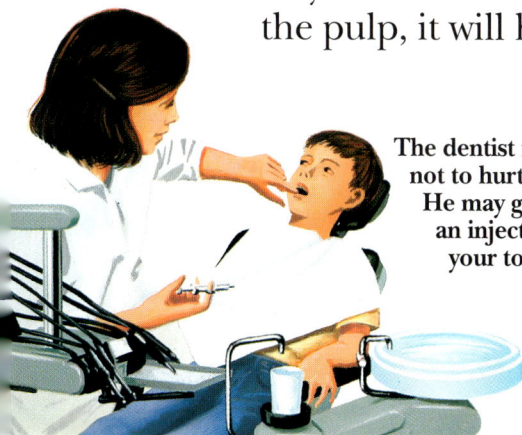

The dentist is careful not to hurt you. He may give you an injection so that your tooth goes numb.

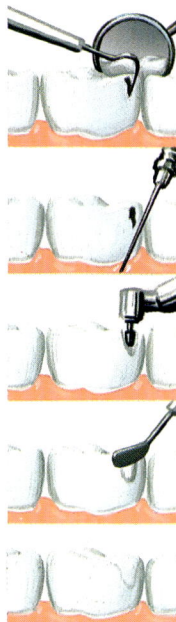

Which would you like best? A glass of milk, 30 grams of cheese or a large cabbage? All these contain the same amount of calcium.

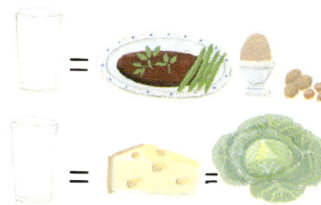

How should you brush your teeth?

Brush them up and down, away from the gums, front and back, for at least three minutes. Then rinse your mouth well. It's best if you can brush your teeth after every meal, but be sure at least to do them after breakfast in the morning and before you go to bed at night. Then you will brush away food which builds into plaque*, as well as germs which could attack the dentine and damage it.

Your teeth, like your bones, grow till you are about eighteen. What you eat will make a difference to how strong your teeth are. Eat plenty of fresh vegetables, as well as milk and cheese for their calcium.

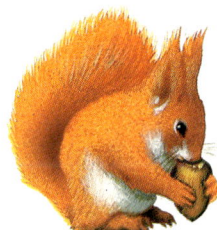

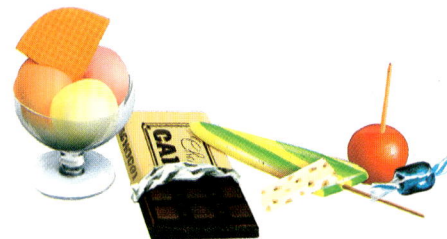

Be careful what you bite – your teeth aren't as strong as a squirrel's!

Biting thread, and crunching sweets and ice lollies are all bad for your teeth.

Sugar is the enemy of healthy teeth!

When sugar mixes with saliva, it turns into acid which eats into the enamel and makes holes. It's fine to eat sweets occasionally, but always brush your teeth straight after you have eaten or drunk anything sugary.

Which are the best things to eat?

If you are going to grow up healthy, you need lots of different foods every day.
You couldn't survive if you only ate one thing all the time, like cake and Coca-Cola. Scientists have shown that the meals we eat during one day should contain at least one food from each of these six groups. Don't forget, we should also drink about ten glasses of water a day.

Meat, fish, eggs (1), and dairy products (4) are building blocks for our balanced diet.

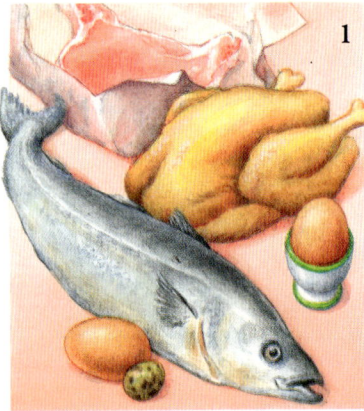

These foods are all proteins and they are vital for the healthy development of your body. Every living part of you needs them if it is to grow and mature properly. Meat gives you iron for your bones and muscles. Fish gives you essential fatty acids, and minerals like magnesium and phosphorus. Dairy products provide calcium for healthy bones. Vitamins are very important while your body is growing and forming. There are lots of vitamins in fruit and vegetables (3).

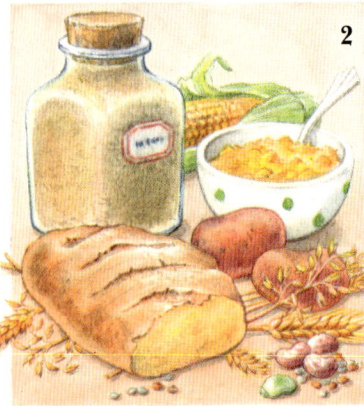

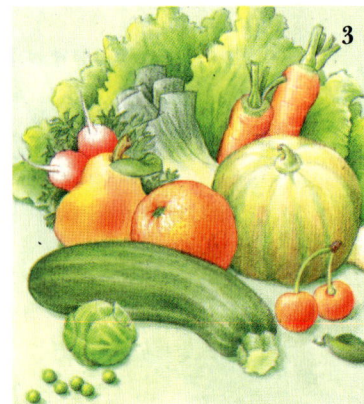

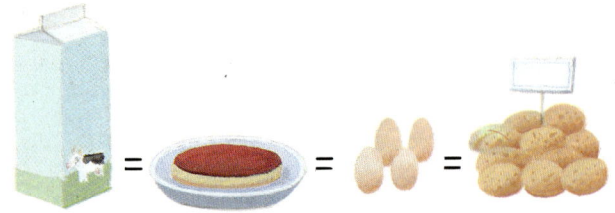

There is as much protein in a litre of milk as there is in a steak, four eggs or a kilo and a half of potatoes.

Carbohydrates: the fuel foods
Foods containing sugar (6), provide us with a boost of energy. We need them, but too many of them can make us fat. Cereals, pulses and starchy foods (2) release energy more slowly throughout the day.

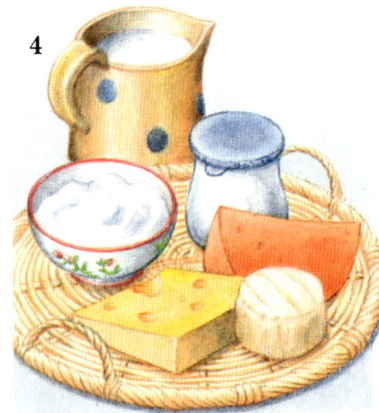

Animal and vegetable fats (5) are harder to digest than carbohydrates, but produce twice as much energy.

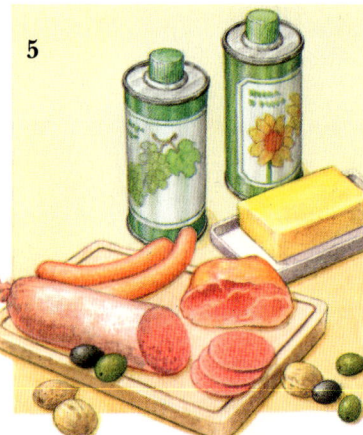

Different people have different needs.
A man, a woman and a child do not all need the same amount of food each day. If you are playing in a football match, you will need more food than if you are spending the afternoon in front of the television. Physical exercise uses up energy fast.

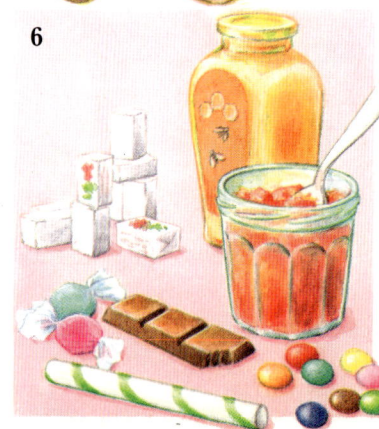

What good does good food do?

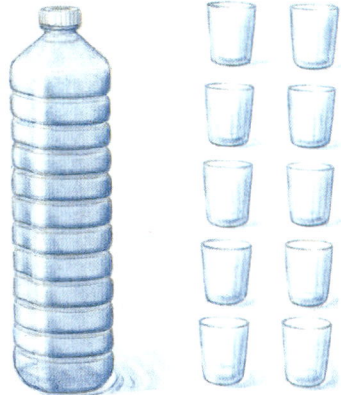

About 70% of your body is made up of water. That's why it is very important to drink water every day: about one and a half litres, that's ten glasses.

A good breakfast is an important start to the day!

Perhaps you eat a cooked breakfast... Breakfast foods vary in different countries, but a healthy breakfast should contain milk or dairy products, cereal or bread, and fruit or fruit juice for their vitamins.

Each vitamin has an important role to play.

Apart from Vitamin D, your body is not able to produce vitamins for itself. You have to eat different foods to obtain them. Vitamin A is important for growth and resistance to infection, and for healthy skin and eyes. There are more than twelve kinds of Vitamin B. They help our nerves, muscles and our digestive system to work properly. They are useful in producing red blood cells and absorbing sugar. Vitamin C helps us fight disease and keeps our tissues and cells healthy. It can be easily destroyed by cooking. Without Vitamin D, our bones would be soft and our teeth brittle. It helps our body make use of calcium and phosphorus to keep our skeleton strong.

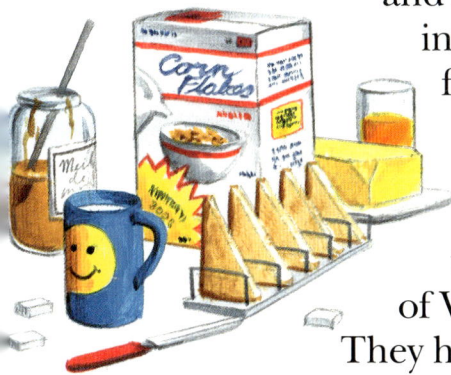

Vitamin E keeps our tissues in good order, so that as we grow older they do not give us too many problems.

Vitamin K plays a vital role in helping our blood to clot.

Where do we find the vitamins that we need?

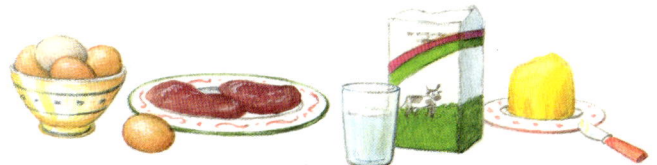

Vitamin A: in liver, egg yolk, butter and milk.

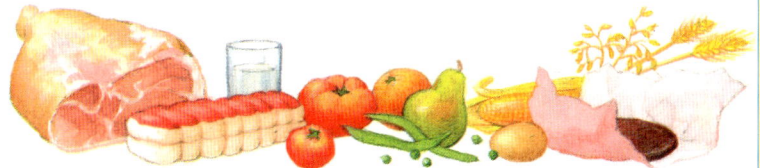

Vitamin B: in fresh meat, egg yolk, milk, meat, cereals, vegetables and fruit.

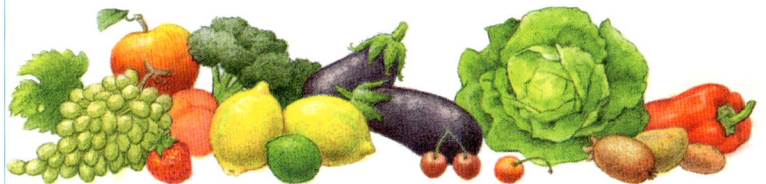

Vitamin C: in citrus fruit, kiwi fruit, potatoes and vegetables.

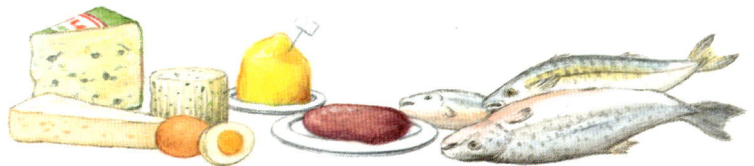

Vitamin D: in liver, egg yolk, butter, oily fish like mackerel and full fat cheese.

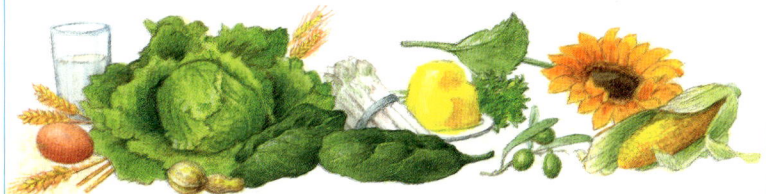

Vitamin E: in milk, vegetable oil, wheat germ and green vegetables.

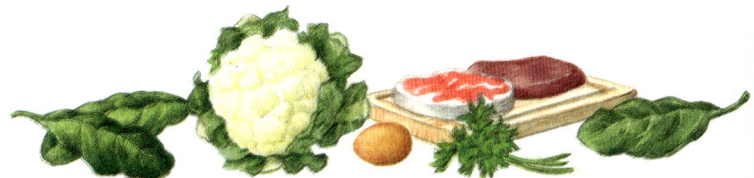

Vitamin K: in liver, eggs, meat, parsley, spinach and cauliflower.

You have been breathing since the moment you were born.

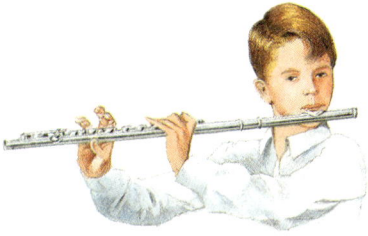

The first thing you did when you were born was to take a great gulp of air: you gave a loud cry, started to breathe and you have been breathing ever since. It is impossible to stop for more than a few moments – otherwise you'd turn blue and suffocate!

It is the oxygen* in the air that supports life on our planet. All our cells need oxygen. The respiratory system is the body's way of breathing and supplying its cells with oxygen.

The respiratory system is like an upside-down tree with its branches in the lungs.

The trunk is the windpipe, the main branches are the bronchi, then come the smaller branches, the bronchioles, which end in a bunch of leaves, delicate air sacs called alveoli. You breathe air in through your nose and mouth. Tiny hairs inside your nose stop dirt and germs going right through the airways.

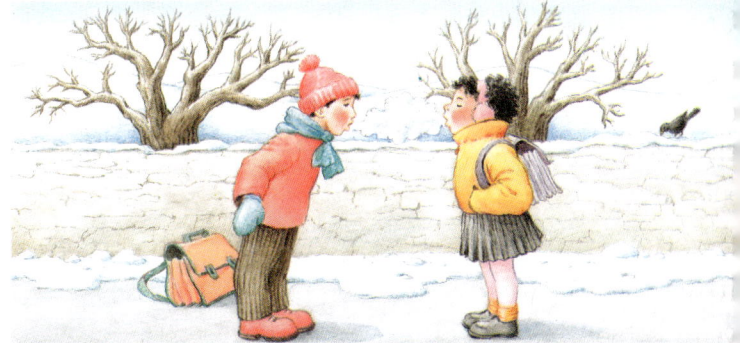

On a cold day you can see your breath, because it is warmer than the air around you and forms a cloud of water vapour.

Down in your lungs, the air meets your blood in the alveoli. The blood takes oxygen from the air, and gets rid of a waste gas called carbon dioxide, which leaves your body as you breathe out again.

How do you speak?

Your vocal cords are stretched across the back of your throat, making a 'voice box'. As you breathe out, the air makes the cords vibrate and produce a sound, just as the cords of a harp vibrate when they are touched.

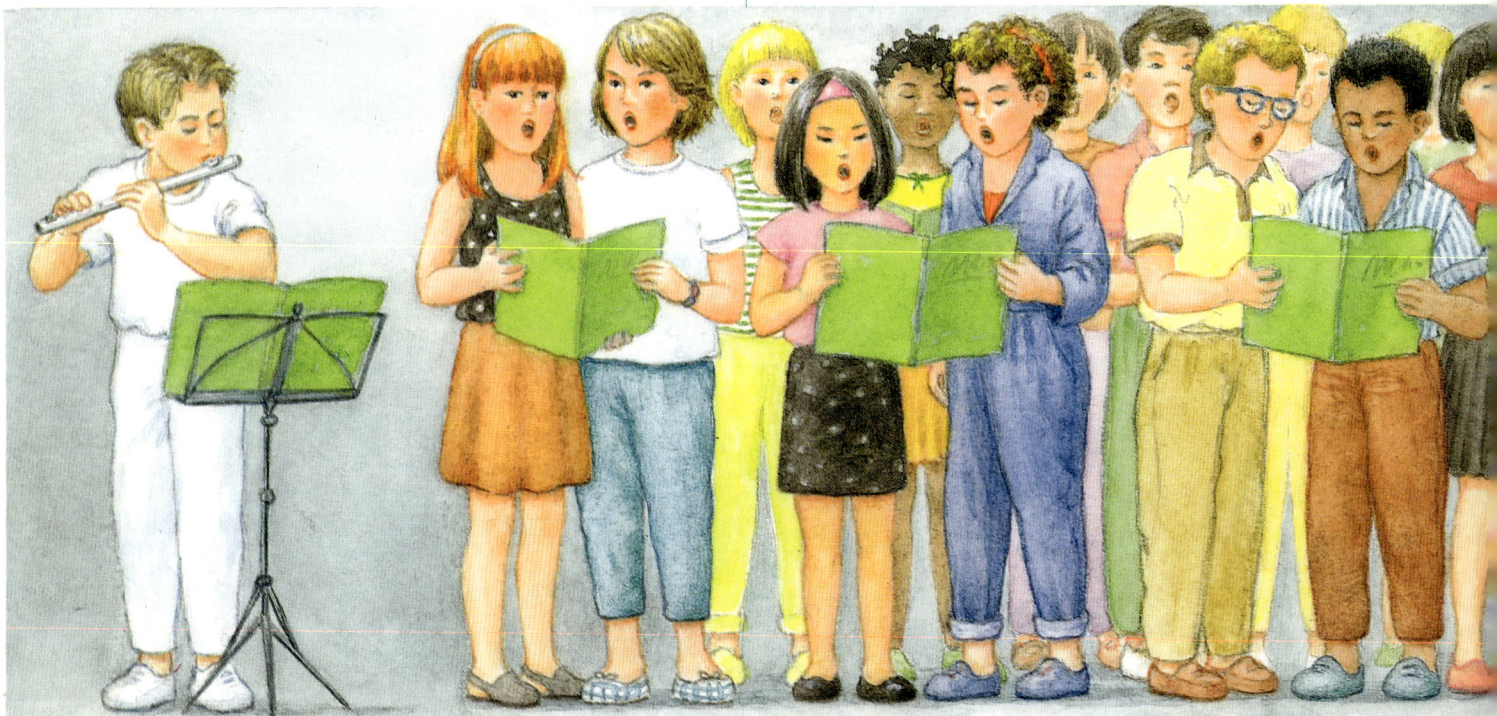

Our lungs have no muscles of their own. Instead, the diaphragm, a big muscle at the base of your lungs, pulls down; your chest expands and air is sucked into the lungs. The diaphragm relaxes and arches up as you breathe out. You breathe in two time: in, out, in, out. You normally breathe without thinking about it, but you can make yourself take deeper, faster breaths.

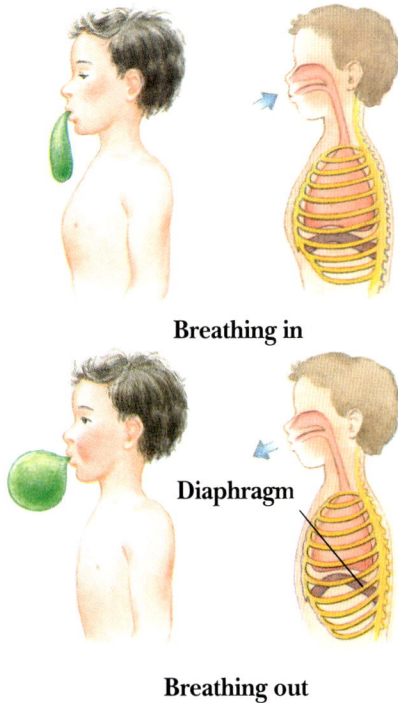

Breathing in

Diaphragm

Breathing out

What are hiccups?
Hiccups are short, sharp and very sudden breaths of air. The diaphragm contracts in jerks, making you gasp.

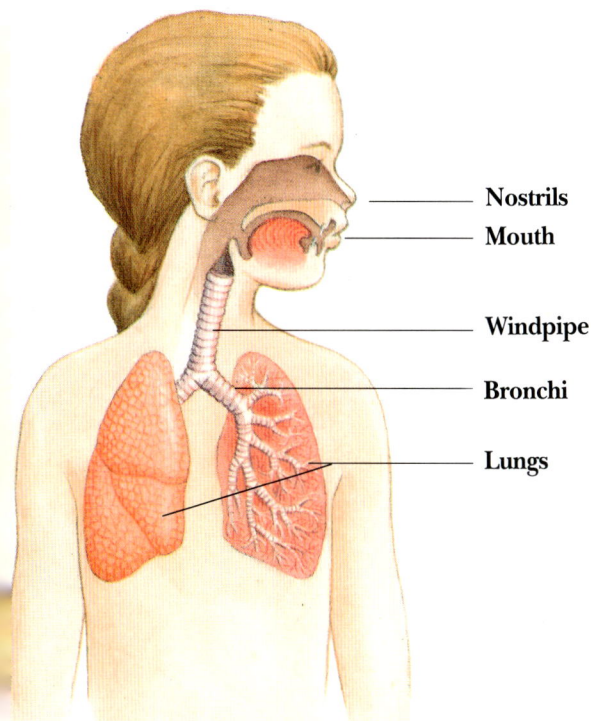

Nostrils

Mouth

Windpipe

Bronchi

Lungs

Colds, sinusitis, bronchitis, pneumonia...
Sometimes it's difficult to breathe and swallow. Your nose is blocked and runs all the time, your voice is hoarse and you're coughing... These are all infections in different parts of the respiratory system. Usually they get better on their own, or with the help of medicine, but if you have pneumonia, or another serious illness you have to go to hospital.

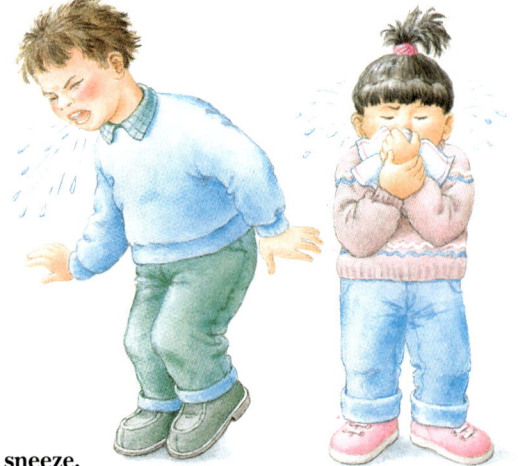

When you cough and sneeze, you are getting rid of germs.

Allergies* can be painful and irritating.
At certain times of the year, especially in the spring, some people can't stop sneezing and their eyes are red and streaming. We say they are suffering from hay fever. In fact, they are allergic to the pollen produced by certain plants. Allergies to dust, feathers, fur and cigarette smoke all set off the same symptoms.

"Government Health Warning!"
Smoking cigarettes can damage your lungs and lead to serious illness. Let's hope you will never give it a try!

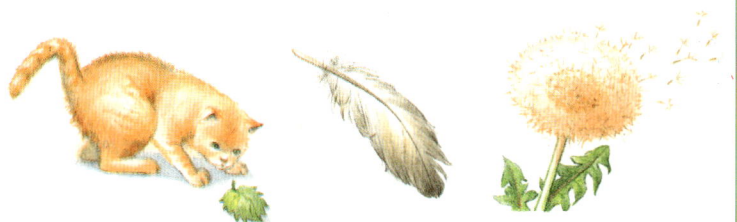

A heart for life

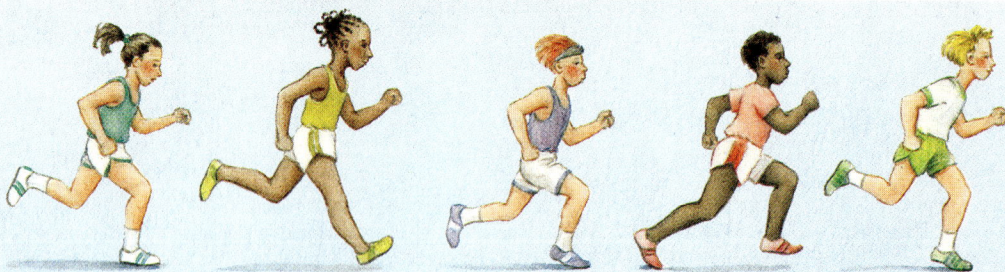

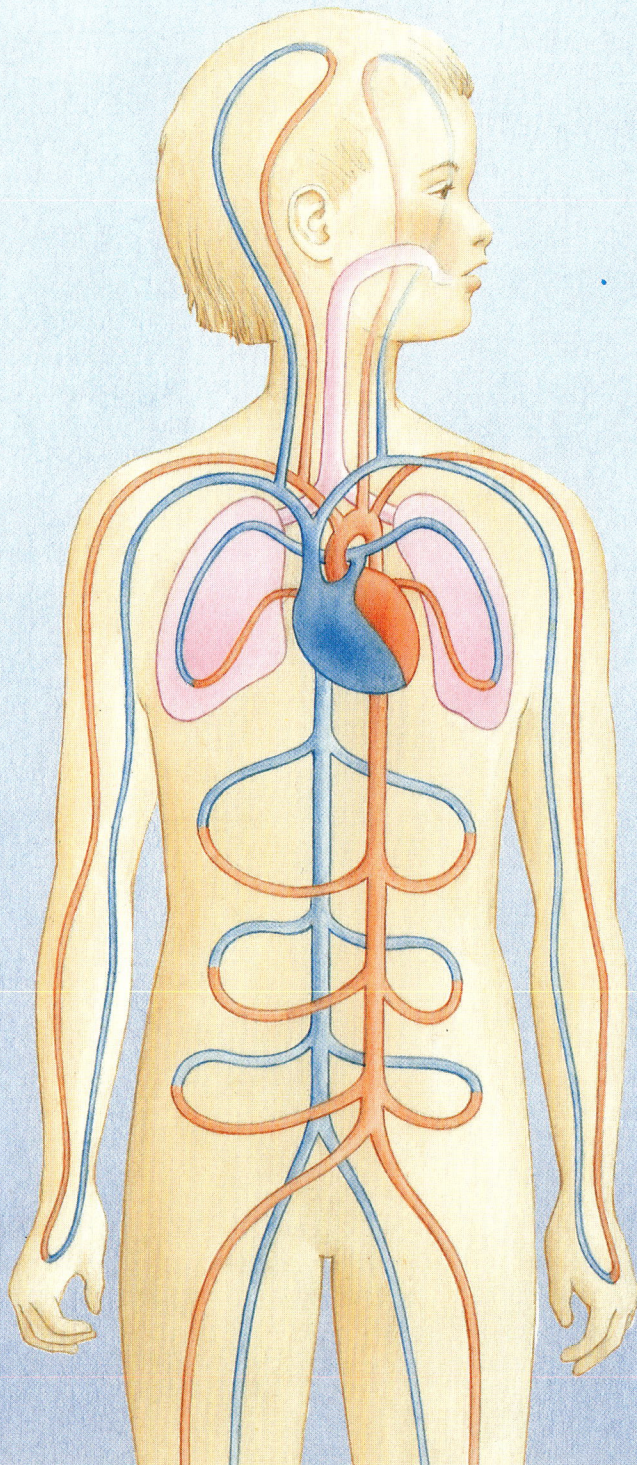

Your heart is the engine of your body. When your heart stops, you've reached the end of your life. That's why your heart is so precious. Yet it's not very big: it's a hollow muscle, just about the size of your fist.

Your heart beats non-stop in your chest. It pumps, then rests, pumps, then rests, about seventy times a minute. As it works, the heart drives the circulatory system.

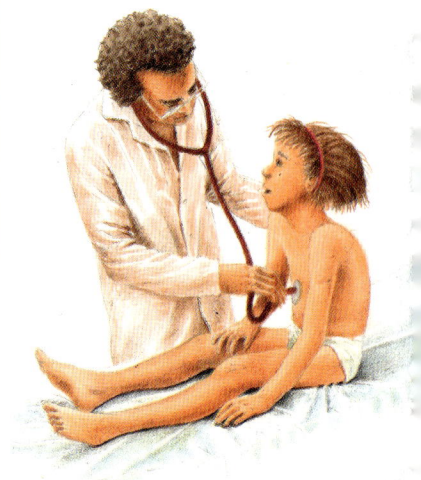

A doctor can listen to your heartbeat through a stethoscope.

You can feel your heart beat faster if you have a big surprise, or if you're excited or frightened. The rhythm speeds up when you are active, and slows down when you are asleep.

The cardiovascular system: the arteries are shown in red, the veins in blue.

Kilometres of blood vessels

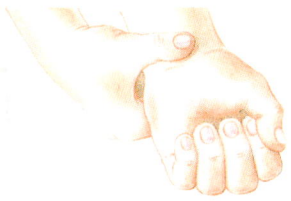

When you take your pulse, you can feel the throb of your heartbeat.

The heart has four chambers: two small ones at the top, called atria, (just one is an atrium), and two larger ones at the bottom, called ventricles.

The heart is divided into two separate parts.

The left side pumps bright red, oxygen*-filled blood right through your body. The right side takes in 'used' blood carrying the waste gas carbon dioxide and sends it to your lungs. Fresh blood and the 'used' blood never get mixed up.

Your heart pumps blood right through your body to your finger-tips.

It goes round in the blood vessels, tubes which can bend and which grow tinier the further they are from your heart, until they are microscopic.

There are two types of blood vessels: arteries and veins.

Arteries, shown in red, carry oxygen-filled blood from the heart to all the cells in our bodies.

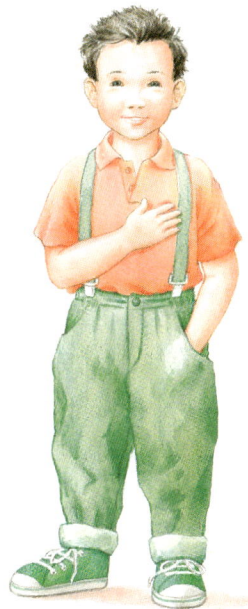

The heart

Superior vena cava

Right pulmonary artery

Right atrium

Right ventricle

Inferior vena cava

Aorta

Left pulmonary artery

Left atrium

Left ventricle

Aorta

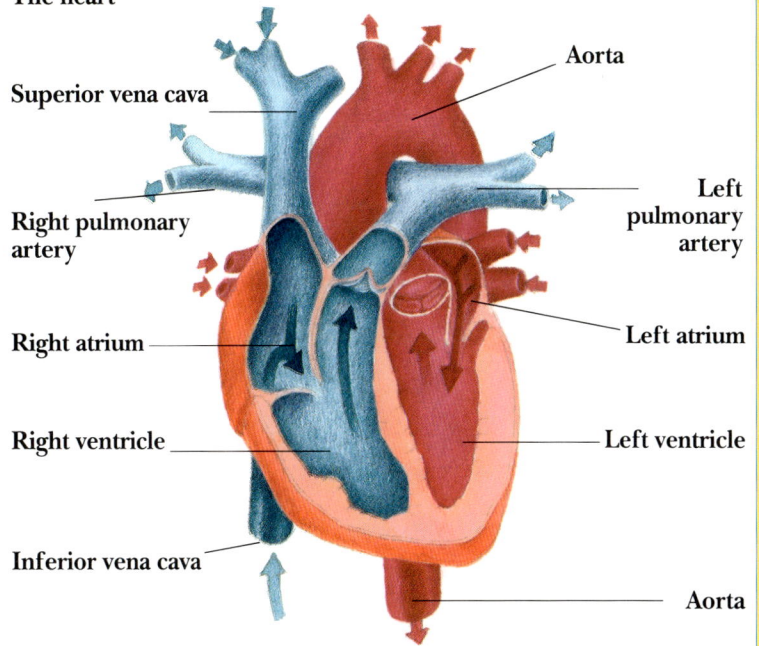

Veins, shown in blue, carry used blood back to the heart and on to the lungs, where it will get rid of carbon dioxide gas. The blood system is like a one-way traffic system: blood goes round in only one direction, valves stop it doubling back.

The heart is fed by two little arteries, the coronary arteries.

They measure only a few millimetres in diameter. These tiny vessels can sometimes get blocked, often as an effect of too much tobacco or cholesterol*. The heart can't go on pumping: the person has a cardiac arrest, or heart attack, and it is very serious. We can help avoid heart disease by not smoking, and not eating too many fatty foods.

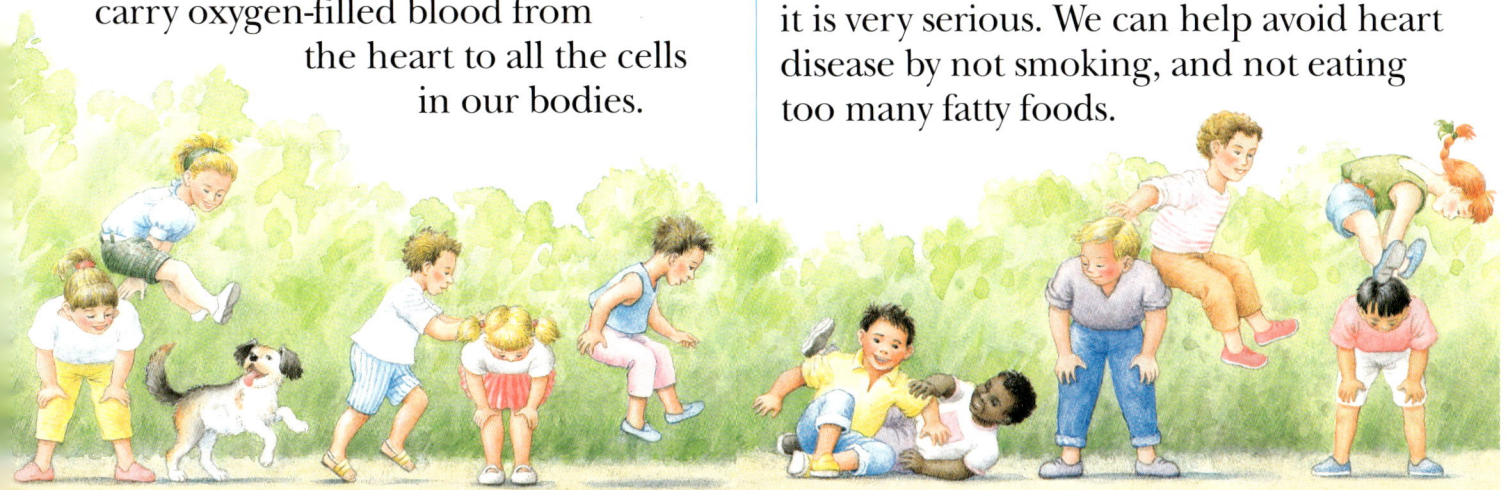

Red blood cells carry oxygen around your body.

When you cut yourself, blood trickles out.

You have about three litres of blood in your body; a grown-up has about five litres. Blood is red and slightly sticky. It is made up of a clear liquid called plasma, in which thousands of tiny cells move about. Some are red blood cells, some are white blood cells and some are platelets.

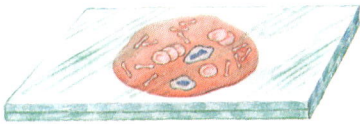

A drop of blood on a microscope slide

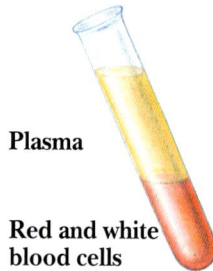

Plasma

Red and white blood cells

There are about sixteen thousand billion red cells in your blood. No wonder you can only see them under a microscope, they're so small!

Each cell has a job to do.

Blood cells are made by bone marrow in the centre of your bones. Each blood cell lives for only three months, so your marrow works non-stop to make new ones.

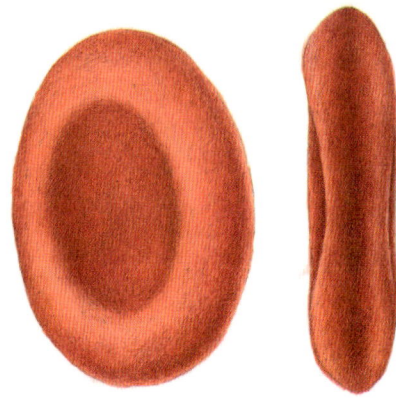

Cross section of a red blood cell, (magnified 8,000 times). Red blood cells get their colour from a substance called haemoglobin, which is the body's oxygen carrier.

What do red blood cells do?

They form a transport system! They carry oxygen* from the lungs to all the body's cells. Every organ is made up of millions and millions of cells. The red blood cells then carry carbon dioxide back to the lungs.

What do white blood cells do?

They are the infection fighters! If you fall ill, they multiply rapidly and set off to attack the germs.

Specially equipped vans stop in town centres so that anyone who wants to give blood can do so. Hospitals need stocks of blood for operations and other emergencies.

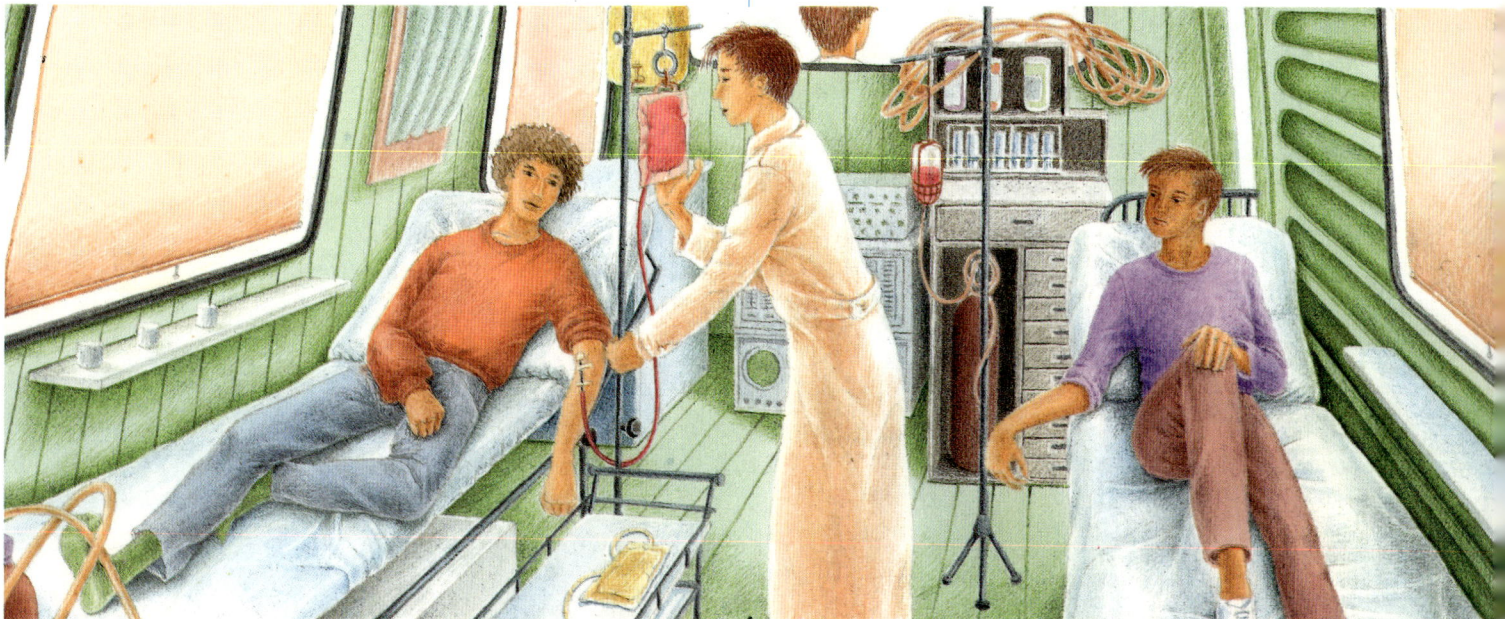

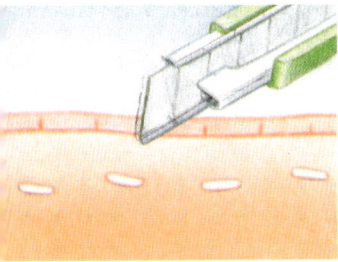

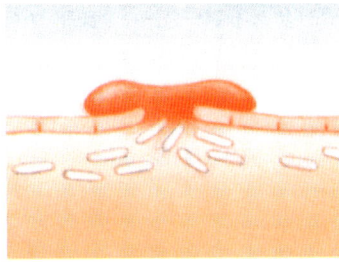

Platelets collect around a wound to form a clot.

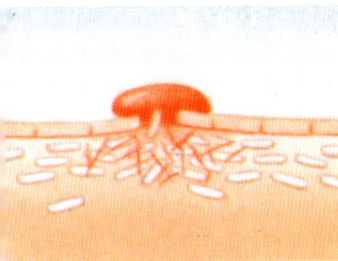

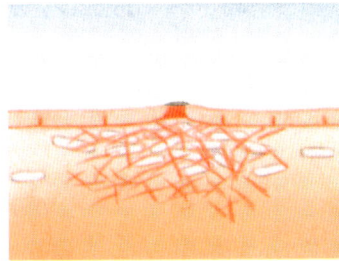

Underneath the clot, special cells repair the damage.
After a few days, the cut has healed.

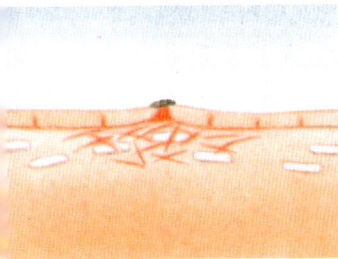

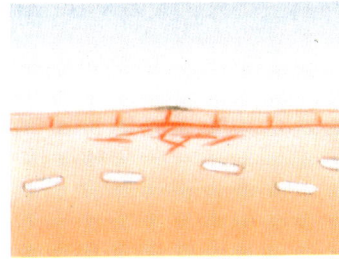

Platelets rush to block a break in a blood vessel.
As soon as you've grazed your knee or cut yourself, platelets get to work to repair the wound. They bind with fibrin to form a clot, a sort of net to hold the blood in. As the clot dries, it turns into a scab. When the wound has healed, the scab falls off, its work is done. You will probably have a little scar for a while.

Don't scratch the scab off if you have a graze. It's there to stop germs getting in.

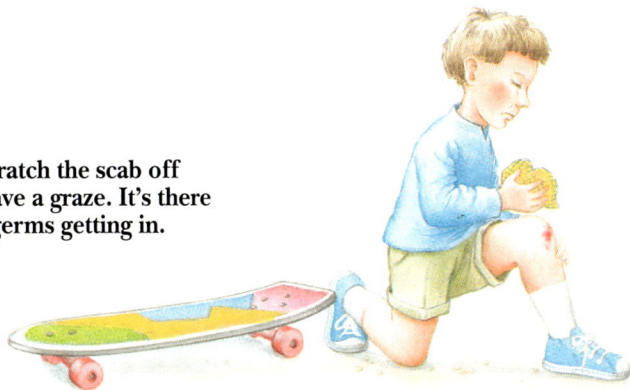

Not everybody has the same type of blood.
There are four different blood groups: O, A, AB and B. It is very useful to know which blood group you belong to. To find out, you have a blood test, and then you will be given a card showing your blood group.

This is important, because not all the different blood groups can be mixed. People with blood group O are called 'universal donors'. They can give their blood to anyone, but can only receive from group O. Group AB can only give blood to others of group AB, but they can receive blood from all the groups: they are universal receivers. Group A can give to A and to AB and receive from A and O. Group B can give to B and to AB, and receive from B and from O. There are also other substances which make matching up blood even more complicated!

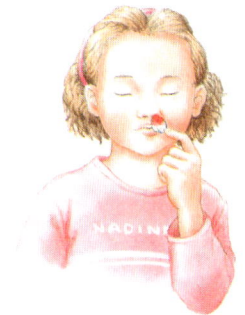

Sometimes you may get a nose bleed.
It happens when a little vessel inside your nose is torn. It looks as if the blood is pouring out, but it's not usually serious!

The lymph system helps to fight disease.
Lymph is a colourless liquid, which travels round the body in lymph vessels carrying white blood cells. Across the path of the lymph vessels are little balls called lymph nodes, which begin to swell up if you have an infection, to make a barrier against any germs.

It's the job of your kidneys to clean your blood.

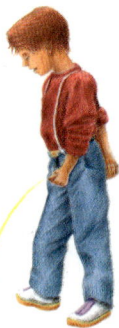

Two kidneys: the perfect filter system

We have seen how the blood collects waste products from the cells of all the organs in the body. If all this waste were allowed to pile up, it would rapidly begin to act like a poison. Your body has to get rid of it: this is the work of your two kidneys. Each is the shape of a broad bean, and a little smaller than your fist.

In the kidneys, blood goes through tiny vessels in contact with millions of tiny filtering units, and the waste products are filtered out just as they would be through a strainer. The waste matter, urea, mixes with water and forms urine; the freshly cleaned blood flows back to the heart.

Where does the urine go?

It collects in the bladder, which is like a little bag. When the bladder is full, nerves send messages to the brain that it's time to empty it. That's when you feel you need to pee. If you wait too long, there may be an overflow! It's important to drink plenty of water to help the kidneys wash away waste.

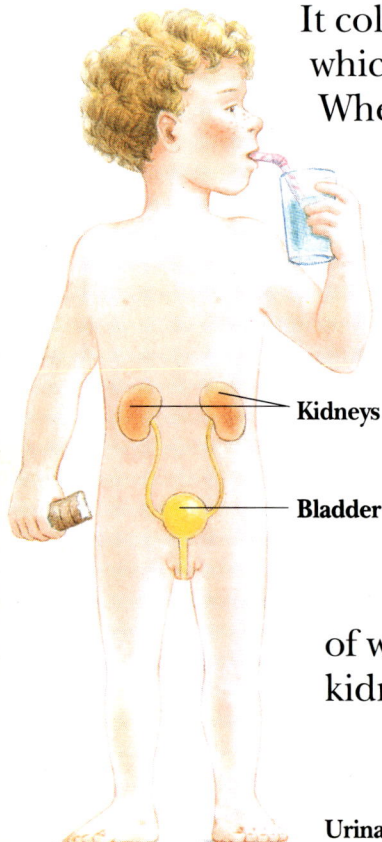

Kidneys

Bladder

Urinary system seen from the front

What's the most obvious difference between a boy and a girl?

Lungs, heart, blood vessels, digestive system: these all work in exactly the same way in both girls and boys.

This isn't true when it comes to the genitals: that's what we call the equipment needed to make babies of our own.

Little girls already have all they will need later on to become mothers: two ovaries to make the ova, a uterus and a vagina. Little boys have two testicles which will hold their sperm, and a penis. But it's not until puberty that these reproductive organs are developed enough to do their job.

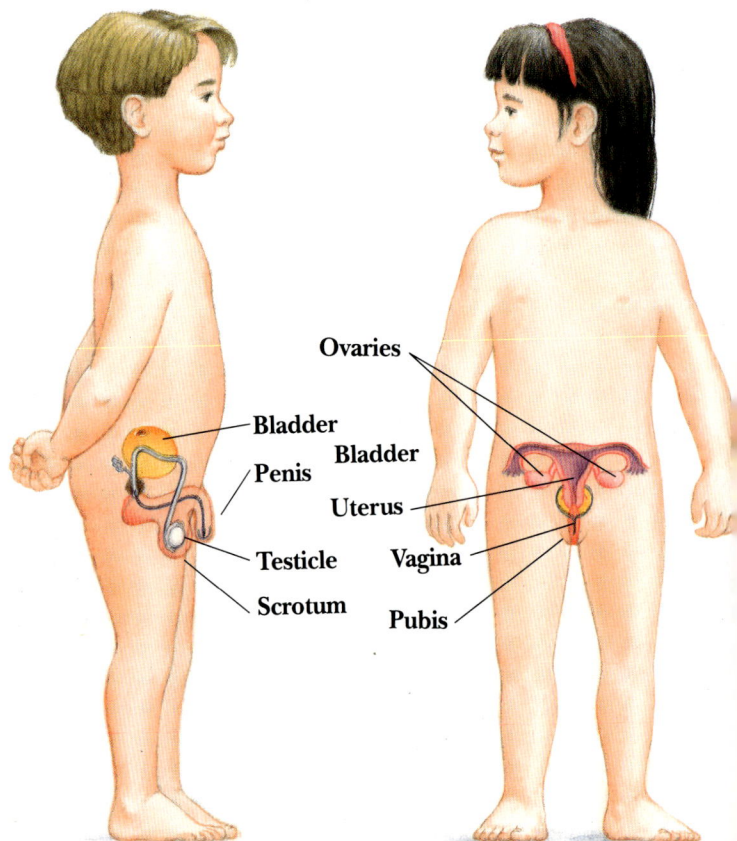

Ovaries

Bladder

Penis

Bladder

Uterus

Testicle

Vagina

Scrotum

Pubis

Puberty is a time of change.
Little boys and girls can't make babies, even if they love each other a lot! Their reproductive organs are not yet ready. Before the ovaries can make the ova, or the testicles the sperm, the body must go through a great change. It happens slowly, over several years, but you can recognize it in all the physical and mental changes that occur between the ages of nine and sixteen. Secondary sexual characteristics appear: with boys, their voices get deeper and they start to grow body hair; with girls, their breasts grow and their periods* start. Teenagers may put on weight and get spots for a while.

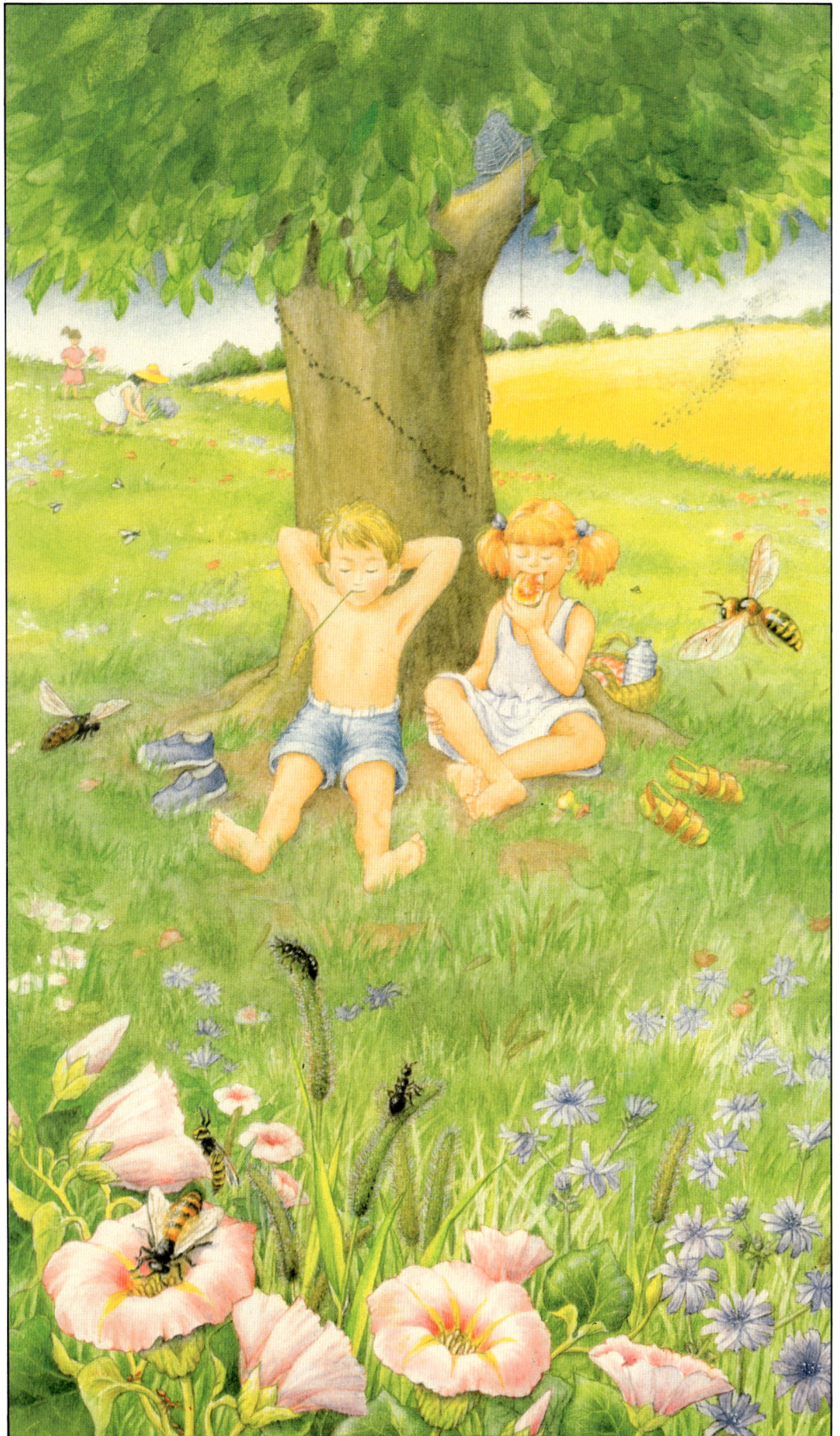

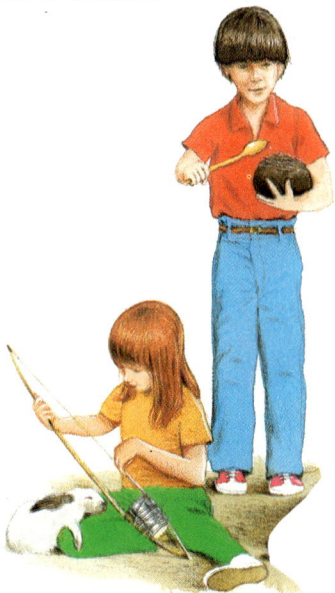

Your skeleton has 208 bones holding you upright.

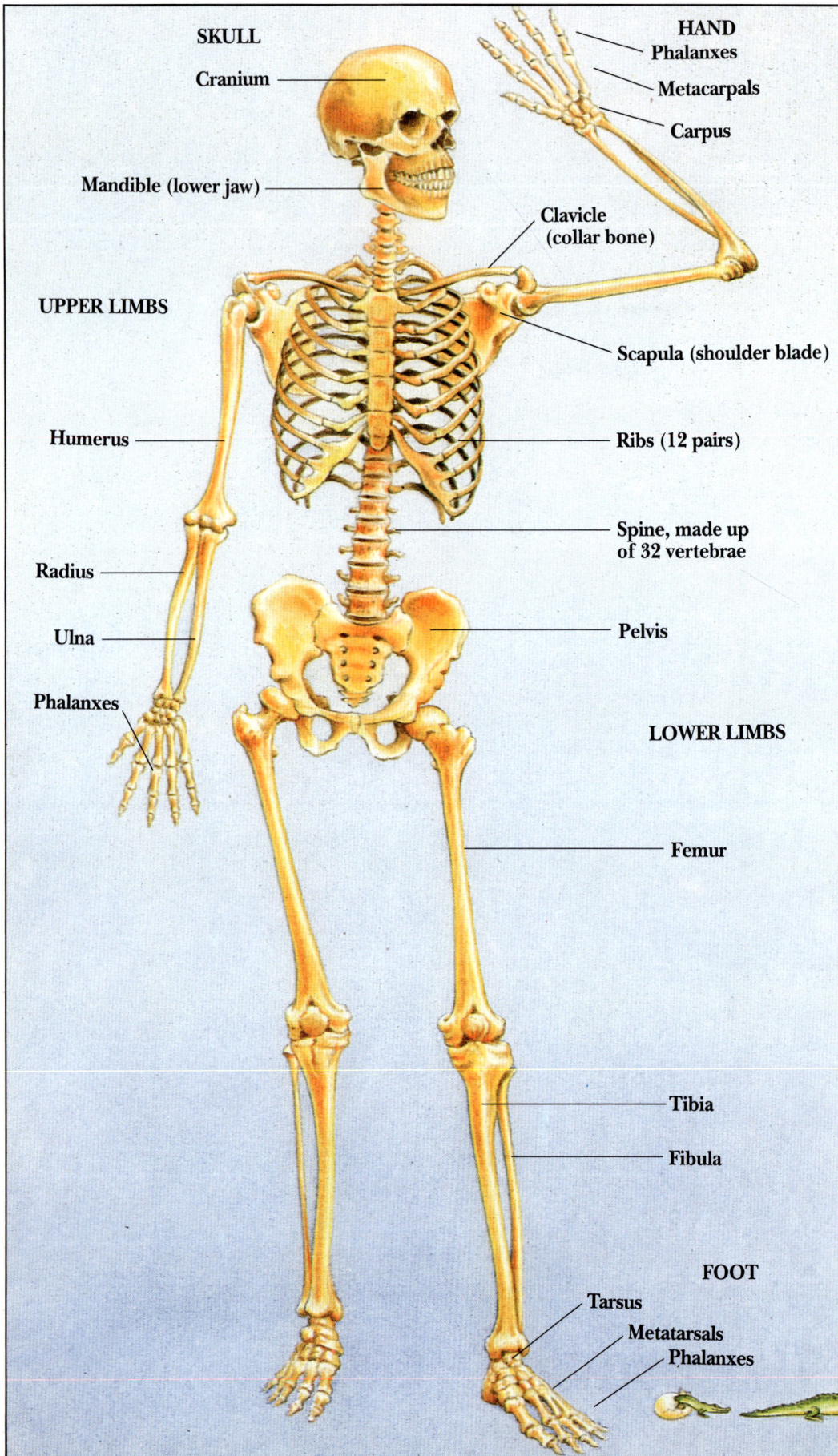

SKULL

Cranium

Mandible (lower jaw)

UPPER LIMBS

Humerus

Radius

Ulna

Phalanxes

HAND

Phalanxes

Metacarpals

Carpus

Clavicle (collar bone)

Scapula (shoulder blade)

Ribs (12 pairs)

Spine, made up of 32 vertebrae

Pelvis

LOWER LIMBS

Femur

Tibia

Fibula

FOOT

Tarsus

Metatarsals

Phalanxes

If you squeeze one of your fingers tight, you will feel something hard: it's a bone. Without a skeleton, you wouldn't be able to stand up.

There are more than two hundred bones in your body, of all shapes and sizes. Some have very funny names: ossicles, scaphoid, coccyx...

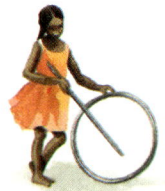

Your tiniest bones are inside your ear; the longest bone is the femur, your thigh bone; others, like your teeth, don't look like bones at all! Some bones form the framework of your body, supporting it and holding it together. Others are there to shield delicate organs: your brain is protected by a solid skull, your heart and lungs are safe behind the buffer of your ribcage...

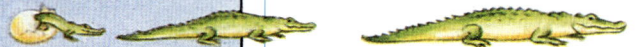

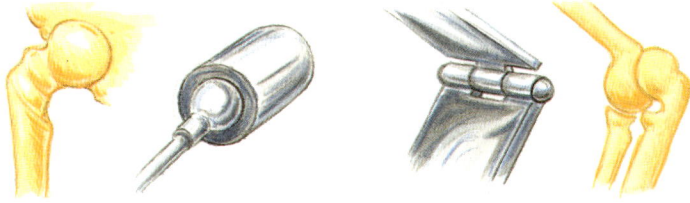

Not all our joints work in the same way. This hip joint is a ball and socket joint: the head of one bone fits into the hollow of another.

This is a hinge joint, which works like the hinge on a door. The elbow and the knee are hinge joints.

Well-oiled hinges to let you bend and twist

Bones are held together at the joints by bands of tissue called ligaments. The bone heads are cushioned with cartilage*, and an oily liquid called synovial fluid keeps the joints moving easily.

Hard bone

Spongy bone

Bone marrow

Cross-section of a femur

A baby's bones are softer than ours.

Gradually, the cartilage they are made from changes and hardens into bone. A little band of cartilage remains at the end of each long bone, allowing it to grow longer and thicker.

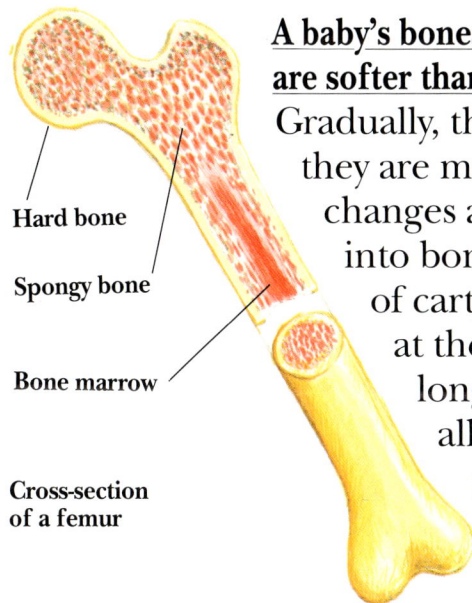

By the time you are an adult, the bands of growth cartilage will have turned into hard bone. Down the centre of the bone runs the marrow, a jelly-like substance where blood cells are made.

Some animals go on growing throughout their whole lives...

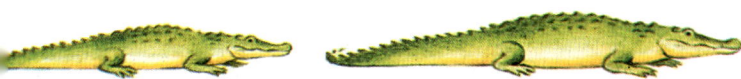

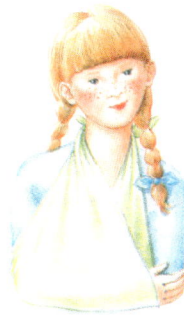

A broken bone can be mended.

You bones are very strong, but they can still break if you have a bad fall. We call it a 'fracture'. The doctor will X-ray the bone to see how badly it is broken.

Sometimes the bones have to be set, or put back in place, to help them mend properly. Then the doctor plasters the broken limb to hold it steady, to give the bone a chance to heal. This can take several weeks.

It's a good thing your bones go on producing new cells; otherwise they could never mend once they had been broken!

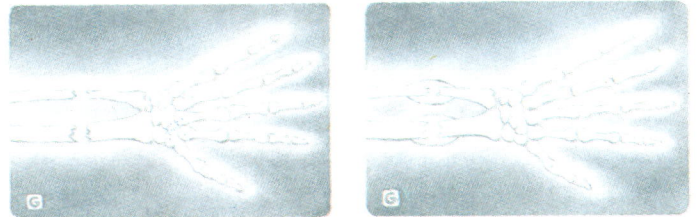

A callus forms where the bone was broken.

When the plaster comes off, you have to do exercises to strengthen the limb that has been hurt.

Bones are made of calcium and phosphorus.

That is why it is important to eat plenty of fish and dairy products, to help your bones to grow and be strong.

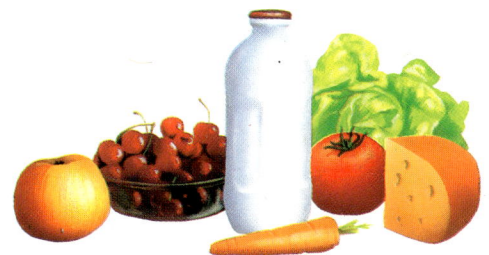

Walking... Running... Jumping

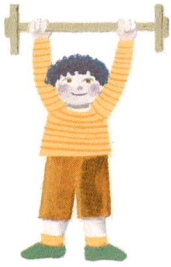

Your bones and muscles make a reliable team!

It would be impossible to have one without the other. Without muscles, your bones wouldn't be able to move.

Muscles are attached to your bones by tendons. They make the bones move by contracting and relaxing: one muscle shortens, the other stretches out.

Your muscles are controlled by nerves.

When your brain gives the order to a muscle to contract, nerves carry a message and the muscle obeys. Muscles cannot push, they can only pull. That's why they often come in pairs and work together to give us a range of movement.

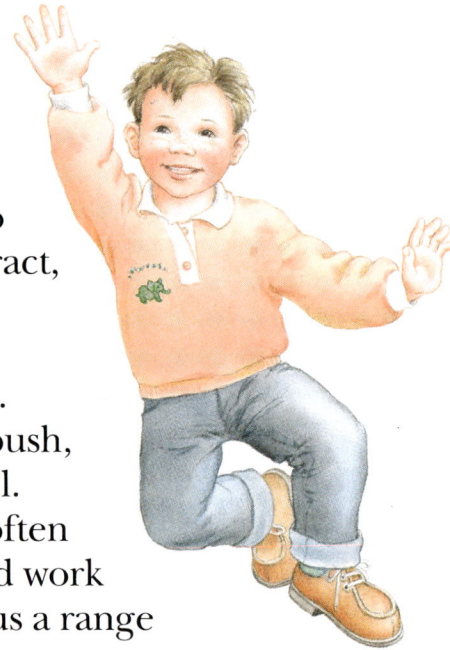

There are more than six hundred muscles in your body.

Some are large, like the ones in your calves or thighs, others are small, like the ones that make your eyes move, or your tongue.

There are several different kinds of muscles.

They aren't all made the same way, or in the same shape. Skeletal, or striped, muscles are the ones we move because we decide to. Some are in the shape of a spindle, like the biceps, some more like a fan, like your back muscles, and some like links, such as your lips and eyelids.

All the muscles which make up the walls of your stomach and intestines are smooth muscle. They work automatically, we can't control what they do even if we think about them.

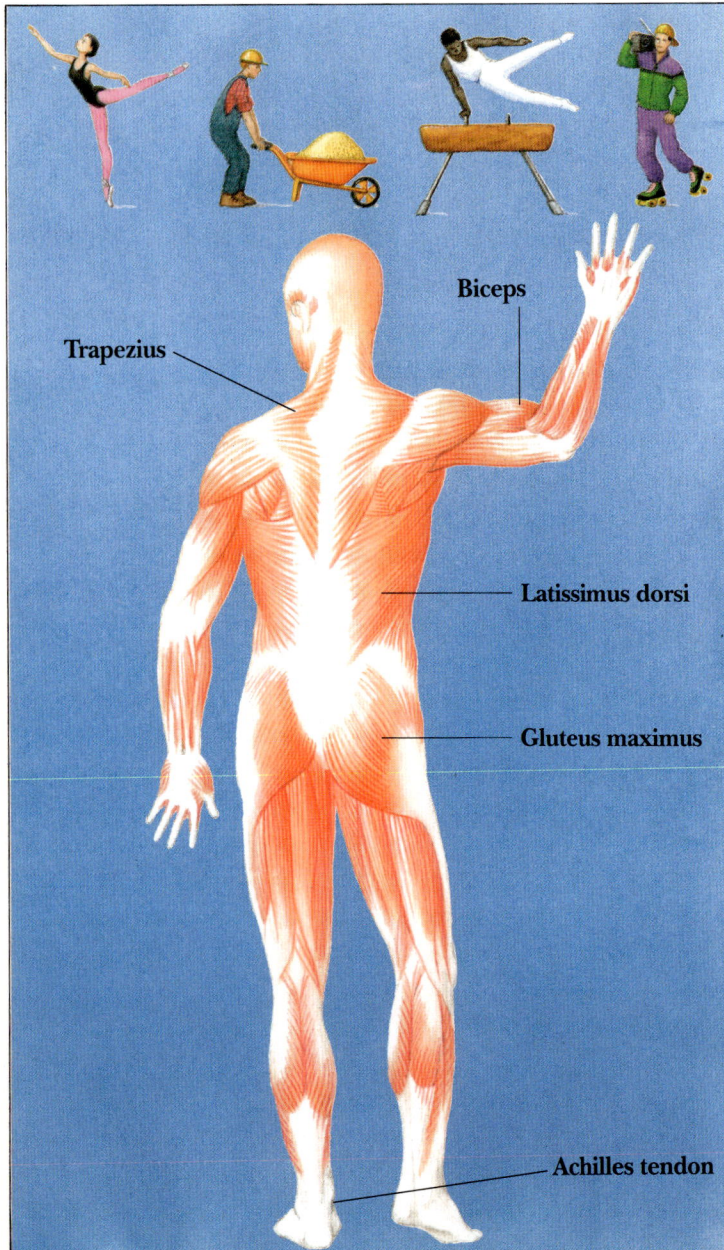

Trapezius

Biceps

Latissimus dorsi

Gluteus maximus

Achilles tendon

Your heart is a very special muscle.

Like all the others, the cardiac, or heart, muscle is controlled by nerves, but it also has an automatic mechanism rather like a battery, which means it can beat on its own as well.

Some baby animals can get up and gallop away the moment they are born.

We don't do that – probably because there isn't a lion round the corner waiting to eat us up!

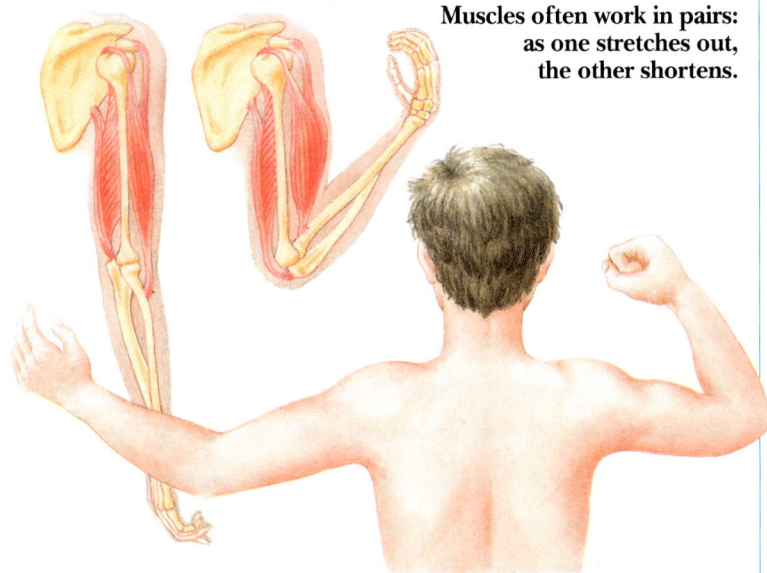

Muscles often work in pairs: as one stretches out, the other shortens.

A new-born baby can't even hold its head up. Gradually, as its bones harden, its muscles grow stronger too and it learns to make different movements.

Muscles need lots of energy if they are to work properly.

Energy comes from the food we eat. As it is digested, the food is broken down into minute particles which are carried by the blood to give energy to all the cells in our muscles.

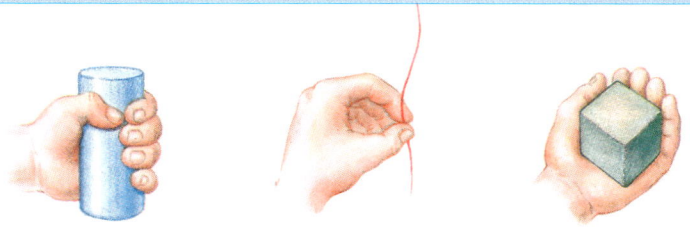

Your muscles enable you to hold and control things. A baby finds it difficult to pick up a thread between two fingers.

The right food will give you energy to play a sport. Drink plenty of water afterwards!

Sometimes your muscles hurt.

Do you ever feel stiff after you have overworked muscles that aren't used to exercise? Or have you ever had cramp, in your calf perhaps: waste products have built up and caused a sharp pain, a warning to rest for a while. If, by accident, you pull a ligament in your ankle or your knee, you will have a sprain.

Taking care of your muscles.

Athletes always warm up before playing sport. It's a very good way of preparing your muscles for the effort you are about to ask of them. They will work better, and you will have less chance of injury.

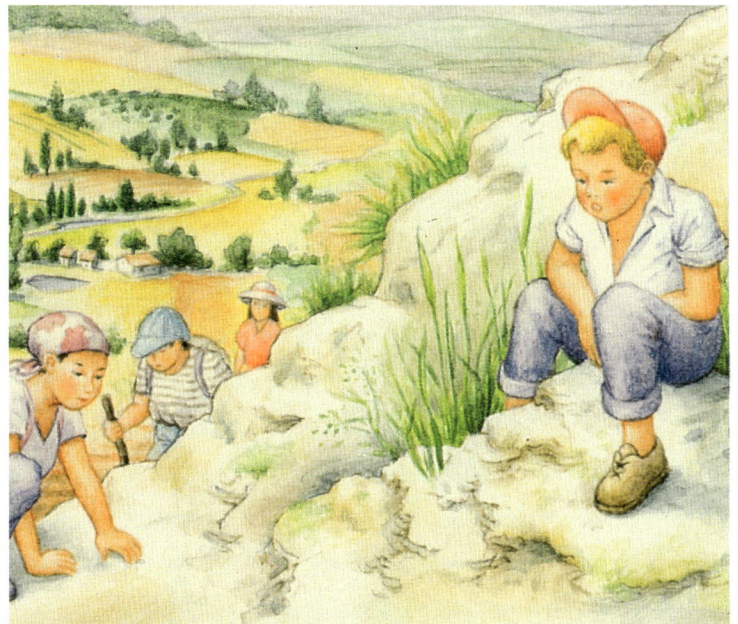

From your head to your toes, your body is wrapped in skin.

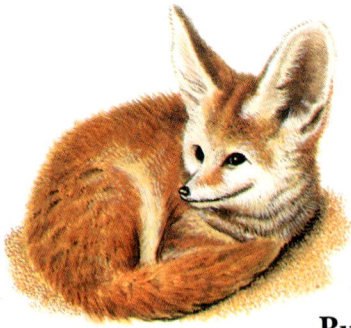

This feels soft, that feels cold – ouch, that hurts! Your skin is full of nerve-endings, which relay what is happening outside your body. But your skin shows up what's going on inside your body too! You blush with embarrassment, you go pale with fright. You're covered in spots, a sign of illness or an allergy.

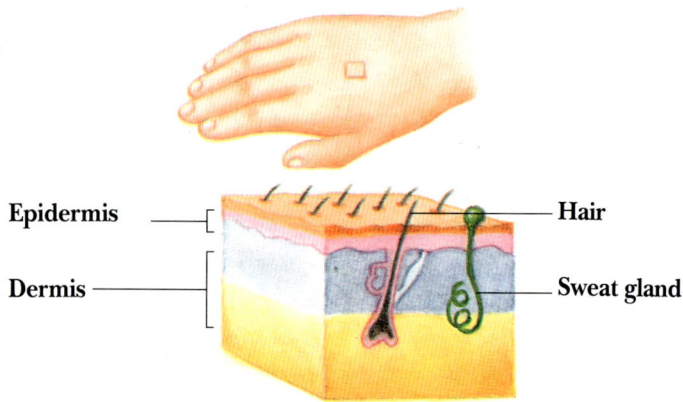

Your skin contains a lot of water. If your body wasn't wrapped in an envelope of skin, the water would run out or evaporate in the air. Then you would look rather like a shrivelled-up prune!

Your skin does not just stop water escaping, it also stops it getting in. It produces a sort of grease called sebum, which makes it waterproof. If it wasn't waterproof, you would swell up like a sponge in the bath!

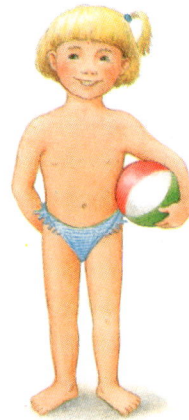

Epidermis — Hair

Dermis — Sweat gland

Your skin is made up of two layers: the epidermis is the very thin top layer, with the thicker dermis underneath. The tiny holes in it are called pores.

Everyone's skin is slightly different.
The pigment* which gives your skin colour is called melanin. Your skin will be darker or lighter depending on the amount of melanin.

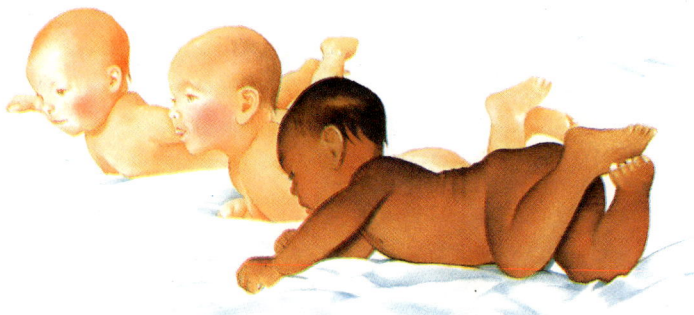

We help our skin do its work by wearing light clothes in summer, and dressing up warmly in winter.

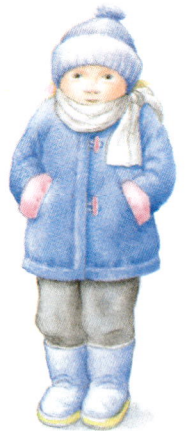

Your skin helps you adapt to hot and cold.
When it's hot, little glands produce sweat, which cools you down as it evaporates. Your blood vessels open up and rise to the surface of your skin to help cool the blood. That's why you look flushed.

When it's cold, your blood vessels contract to keep in heat, and the hairs on your arms and legs stand up: you've got goose pimples!

Skin protects you from germs.
Healthy skin makes a very strong barrier against bacteria.

It's important to look after your skin.

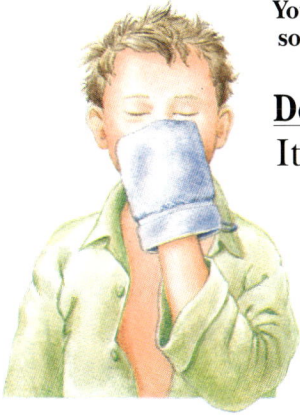

Your face is never covered up,
so it needs a good wash twice a day.

Do you like washing?
It's a good thing to have a bath or a shower every day because dirt and dust stick to sebum. As you rub yourself, you take off the old layer of grease. It's replaced at once with a new one.

Bumps and bruises
Your skin is strong; it's good protection. But accidents happen now and then. It is very important to clean cuts and grazes. If you have a bump, the blood and lymph vessels can be crushed slightly, even if the skin is not broken. Liquid spills out and causes a swollen lump. Special cells in the surrounding tissues help repair the damage. In a few days, the swelling will have disappeared.

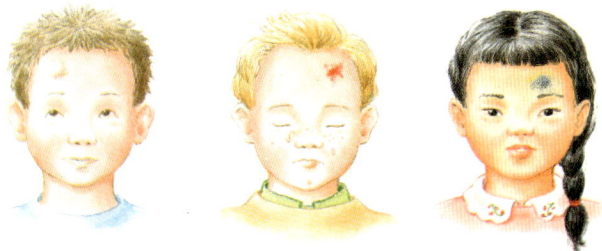

You fall over, and there you are with a bump, a graze or a bruise – and if you're unlucky, all three at once!

The same sort of thing happens when you're bruised. The little blood vessels get crushed, and a pool of blood forms under the skin. Blood vessels mend quickly, and blood soon stops leaking out. Bruises change colour, from dark purple to blue, then yellow, before they disappear.

Be especially careful of burns and scalds!
Boiling water, a hot iron, electricity, a light bulb that's switched on... lots of things around the house can burn you. Our skin can't stand very high temperatures. When you burn yourself, you lose your protective layer of skin and you're in danger of losing your body's fluids. All burns are painful.

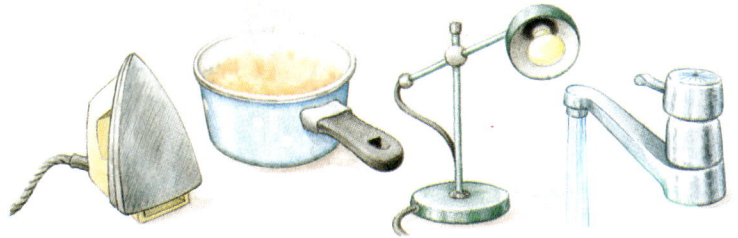

A first degree burn makes your skin turn red; a second degree burn causes blisters; a third degree burn starts to destroy the skin, turning it blackish.

Sun burns too!
You need to be careful not to get sunburned, especially if you have fair skin. Normally, your skin protects itself from the sun by producing more melanin. Your skin goes brown and has greater resistance to the sun's rays. A protective cream or lotion gives your skin an extra barrier for the first days in the sun. Scientists now know that too much exposure to strong sun is very harmful for years to come, and can cause skin cancer. So, though it's nice to tan – be wise!

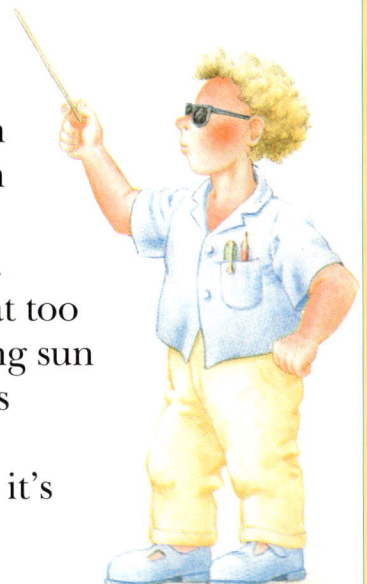

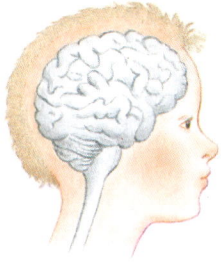

What controls and organizes all the different body systems? What enables you to have feelings, thoughts, ideas? The nervous system, highly perfected and complex, made up of the brain, the spinal cord and 43 pairs of nerves. The brain itself is made up of the cerebrum, the cerebellum and the brain stem.

Your brain is made up of billions of nerve cells, called neurones.
Cells like these are also found in the spinal cord and the nerves. Neurones are shaped rather like tiny stars, with lots of elongated arms trailing in all directions to pick up messages from other cells.

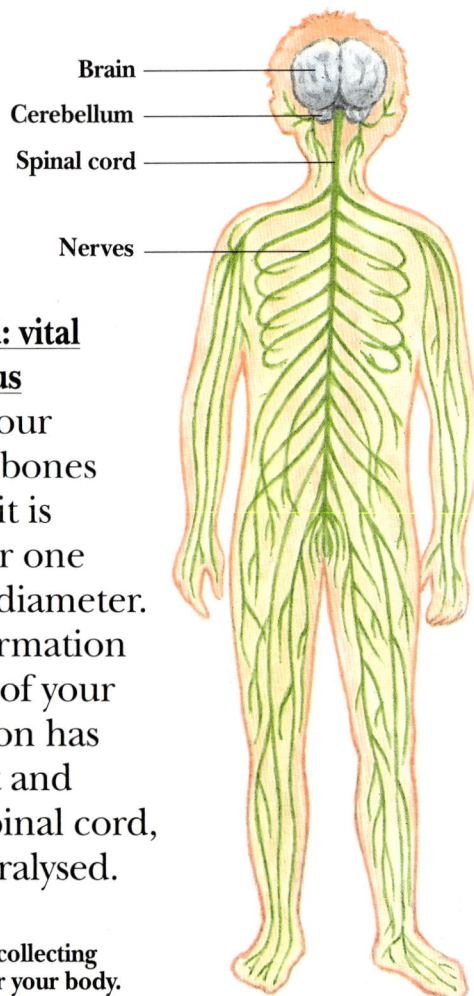

Brain
Cerebellum
Spinal cord

Nerves

Your spinal cord: vital and very precious
Protected by your vertebrae, the bones of your spine, it is a cord just over one centimetre in diameter. It collects information from all levels of your body. If a person has a bad accident and breaks their spinal cord, they will be paralysed.

Your spinal cord is like a central cable, collecting messages from all over your body.

A baby is born with all its neurones already in place.
While it was still in its mother's tummy, it was acquiring millions of new neurones every minute, so it has hundreds of billions in reserve. This is just as well, because neurones do not renew themselves, and you start to lose them from the age of twenty onwards. If a nerve cell is destroyed, it cannot be replaced.

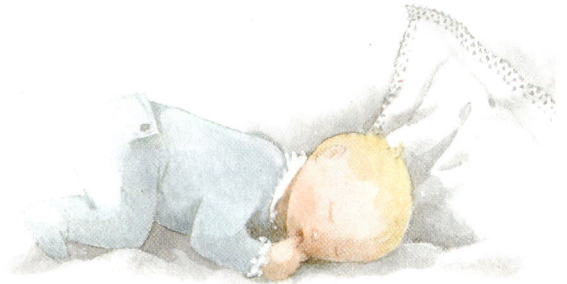

It has taken billions of years for our brain to evolve into such an extraordinary, ultra-perfected organ. Humans beings are the only creatures to have such a high-performance brain.

Cradled safely inside your skull, the cerebrum is divided into two hemispheres: left and right.
Each is wrapped in a sort of grey matter called the cerebral cortex.
When you are young, the cortex is smooth. As you grow older, it creases and the surface begins to look rather like a walnut.

Make your two hands into fists for a minute, put them one against the other, and you'll have an idea of the size and shape of your brain.

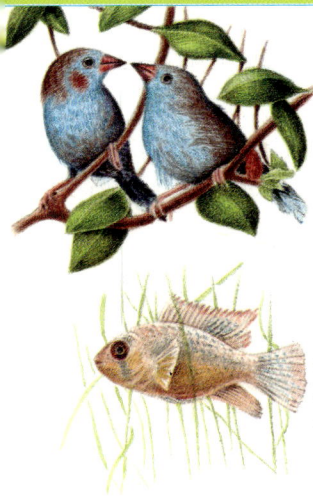

Has anyone ever called you a birdbrain when you've done something silly? That's because animals have brains which are far less developed than yours.

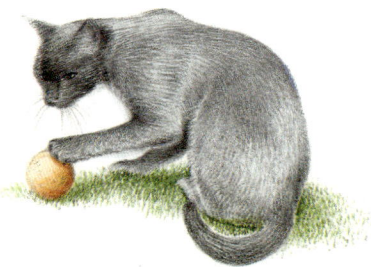

Nerves which stretch for kilometres!

If you think of your brain as the centre of a telephone system, the nerves are the network of telephone lines relaying messages. Sensory nerves carry information from your skin and sense organs to your brain, motor nerves carry messages from the brain to your muscles.

Thousands of messages, or nerve impulses, are circulating round your body all the time.

The brain receives these messages through the neurones in your nerves and spinal cord. It uses neurones to send out instructions too.

Some of these messages are under your control.

The traffic light shows a green man; you know you can cross the road. The phone rings; you pick up the receiver.

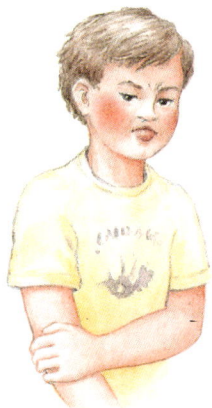

The cube will fit through the square hole: it's your brain which is giving you the instruction.

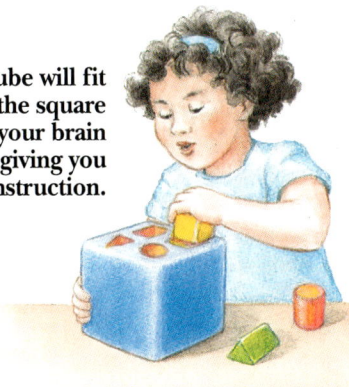

Many messages are independent of your will.

One area of your brain looks after the rhythm of your heart beat, your breathing, your digestion, making sure your glands work, your sleep, your appetite... all those things which happen all the time, without you even thinking about them. If something makes you very frightened, your heart begins to beat very fast and your breath comes in gasps whether you like it or not!

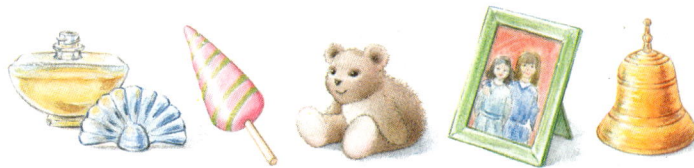

The five senses: smell, taste, touch, sight and hearing are regulated by the brain.

You can make your brain perform better, especially your memory, if you keep it well exercised.

The different zones in the brain:
1. Motor area controlling movement
2. Sensory area
3. Sight
4. Hearing
5. Smell
6. Speech

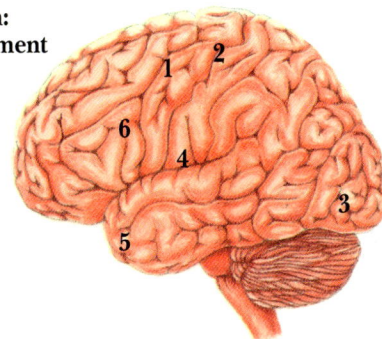

We now know that the cortex is divided into different zones, each specializing in a different set of responses and actions. Each hemisphere receives messages from the opposite side of the body, and also directs the activities of the opposite side.

Your right hand touches something hot: the message arrives in the left hemisphere of your brain, which sends the instruction to take your hand away.

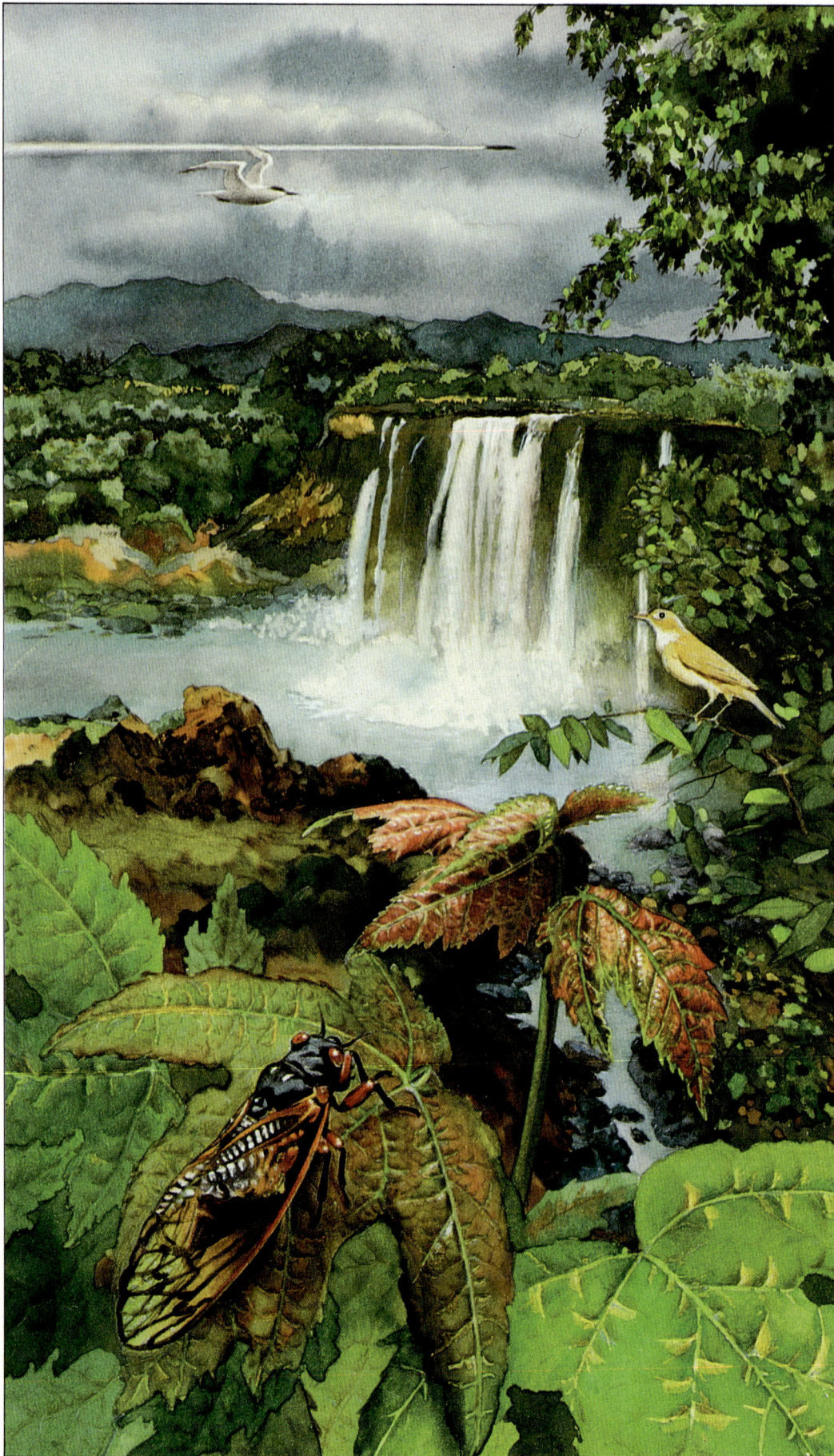

We learn about the world through our senses. Thanks to them, we can get to know the world around us. We can see beautiful landscapes, hear music, taste delicious food, smell the scent of flowers and feel the softness of their petals.

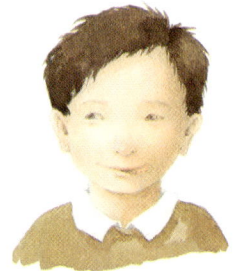

What are the five senses?

Sight, hearing, smell, taste and touch.
Your eyes, ears, nose, tongue and skin are your sense organs.

Each one detects sensations and sends messages to your brain through the sensory nerves. We've seen that each sense has a corresponding zone in the cerebral cortex. Your brain then sends out instructions to your muscles through the motor nerves.

It's up to us to use and develop our senses.

If you do not pay attention to your senses, you may find yourself living in a dull, muffled kind of way.
But if you concentrate on what they tell you, you will find that your body opens up to a world of variety... Your senses will help you get the very best out of life!
If you have lost, or were born without, one of your senses, you've probably developed the others far more than your friends who have all five. A blind person often has a very keen sense of touch and hearing.

Animals have very highly developed senses.
Often, one will be stronger than all the rest.
Birds have little sense of smell, but they are very sharp-sighted. Fish have a very strong sense of smell, and they also have special auditory* organs on their skin which work like ears. Snails use their antennae to taste. A snake collects smell with its forked tongue, which flickers in and out, picking up scents from the air.
Each one uses its sense of sight, touch, hearing, taste and smell in its own particular way.

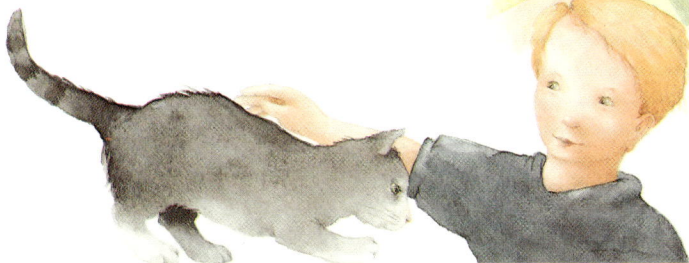

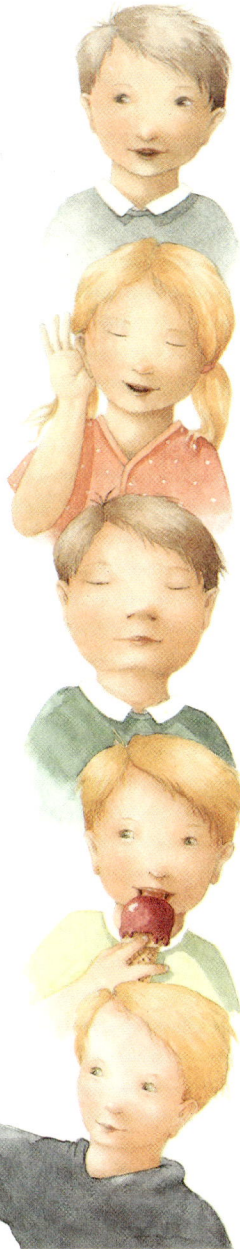

Foxes and dogs can hear sounds out of range of human ears.

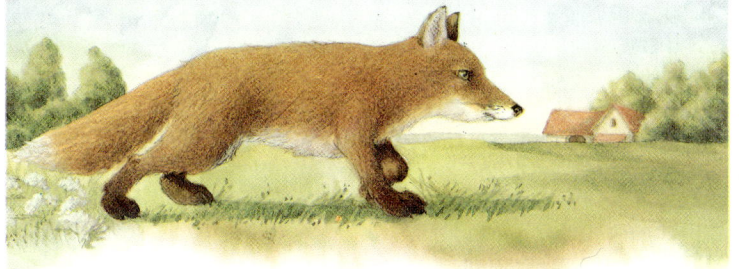

Some animals seem to have a special sense.
Something terrible is going to happen. What can it be? The hens are panicking, the horses trembling, the swallows twittering, long before humans have any idea that something is wrong. Animals are particularly sensitive to vibrations, so that they can judge when there is going to be an earthquake, for instance.
Before flies take wing, they stretch out their antennae to find out how hard the wind is blowing.

A cicada hears through organs on either side of its abdomen.

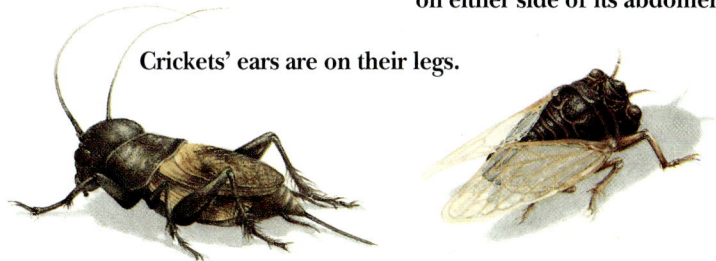

Crickets' ears are on their legs.

Female mosquitoes, which feed on blood, use their antennae to sense the presence of a warm-blooded animal or person from several metres away.
Dolphins and whales, like all cetaceans*, have a sixth sense, sonar. They send out sounds which bounce off the objects around them. The nature and direction of the echo tells them the shape of the object and how far away it is.

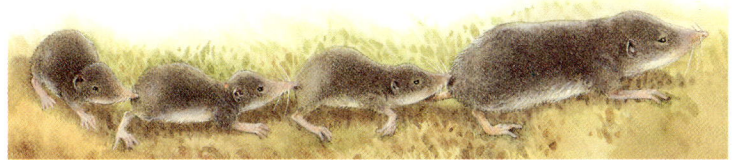

The eye is a very delicate organ.

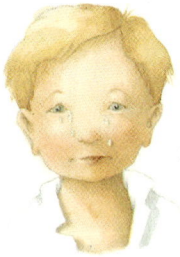

What is an eye?

The eye is a soft globe protected by eyelids. It is set in a cavity called the orbit. Your eyes move a lot, even if you think they are still, and in all directions: they are held in place in the orbit by muscles. Tears wash the eye constantly, keeping it moist. They are spread across the eyeball by the eyelids, which blink about once every ten seconds.

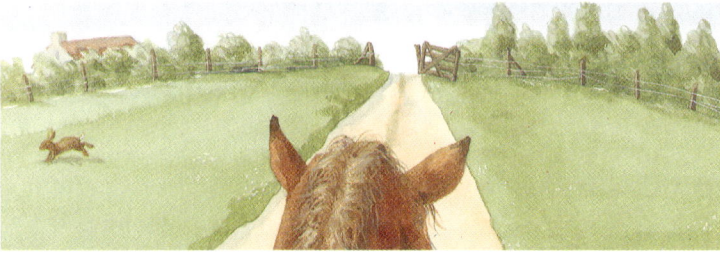

A horse cannot see things which are directly ahead very clearly, but it can see a long way to either side.

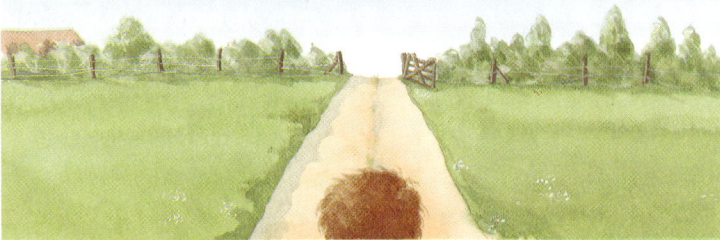

We cannot see as far to the side as a horse can, but we do see more clearly, because the vision of each eye overlaps.

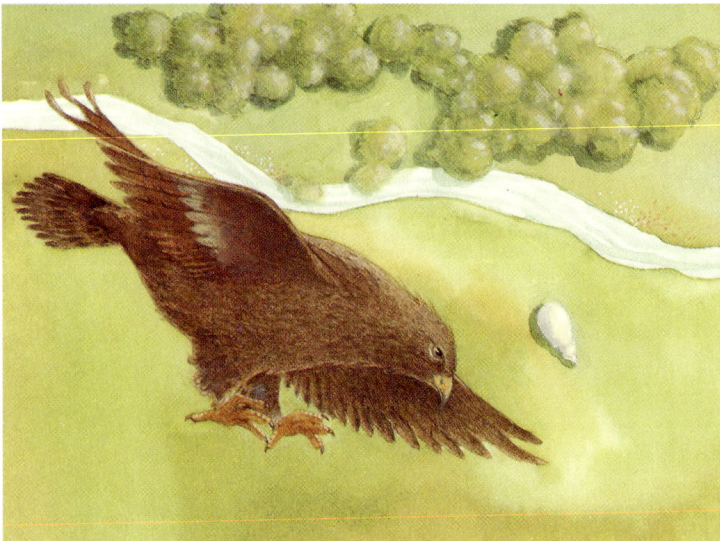

Eagles are very sharp-sighted, and can spot their prey, a mouse for instance, from a great height.

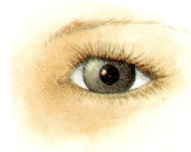

Eyelids and eyelashes protect the eyes.

1. Cornea
2. Iris
3. Pupil
4. Lens
5. Retina
6. Optic nerve

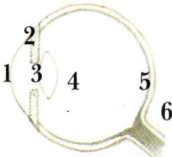

Tears are made by the lacrimal glands just under your upper eyelids. No-one knows exactly why they work so hard when you are sad.

The iris, which can be brown, blue, grey or green, is protected by a transparent membrane* called the cornea. The black dot in the centre of the iris is in fact an opening, called the pupil. The lens behind the pupil changes shape according to whether the eye is looking at things close up or far away; this is called focusing. Light passes through the pupil and the lens, and falls on the retina at the back of the eye.

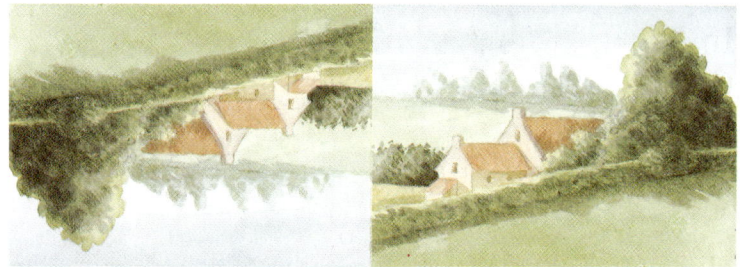

To see things in three dimensions, both eyes need to be working properly.

Information is carried from the retina to the brain by the optic nerve. Your left eye can see a little more to the left, and the right eye a little more to the right. As the lens focuses an image on the retina, it turns the picture upside down. When the brain receives the information, it turns the image the right way up again.

An eye doctor is called an ophthalmologist. He uses a special instrument to see through the pupil to the retina, right at the back of your eye.

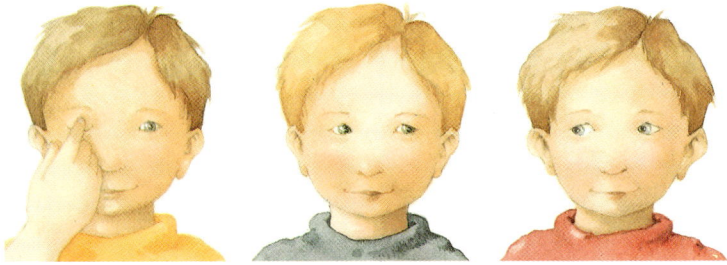

Eyes can move a lot, quickly and in every direction, thanks to the muscles which fix them to the orbit.

Dragonflies have up to 40,000 tiny lenses in each eye. Their eyes cover almost the whole of their heads.

Do you wear glasses?

If you do, it is because your eyes do not work perfectly. If your eyeball is too long, you are short-sighted. You can see things that are near quite clearly, but things that are a long way off look blurred. If your eyeball is too short, you are long-sighted and the opposite is true. Glasses help to focus the image on the retina.
If you are astigmatic, it means that your lens or cornea is an irregular shape, and you will have blurred or double vision.
In fact, no-one's eyes are perfectly round. Older people tend to need glasses because their lenses and muscles aren't as supple as they used to be, and don't work as well. They are usually long-sighted.

If a person squints or looks cross-eyed, it means that one of the eye muscles isn't directing the eye correctly. The problem can often be solved by doing eye exercises, but sometimes an operation is necessary.

Glasses are made for just one pair of eyes.

Your friend's glasses won't be much help to you!
The ophthalmologist has your glasses made up especially for you at an optician. When you are older, you may prefer to wear contact lenses, little round lenses that you learn to put directly on to the surface of the eye.

Insects can see ultra-violet colours which we cannot see.

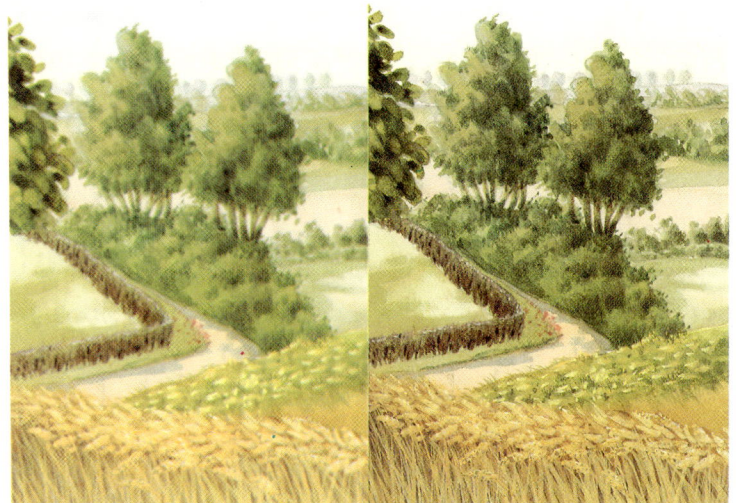

When it is dark, the pupil opens wide to let in as much light as possible. In bright light, though, it shrinks and becomes very small.

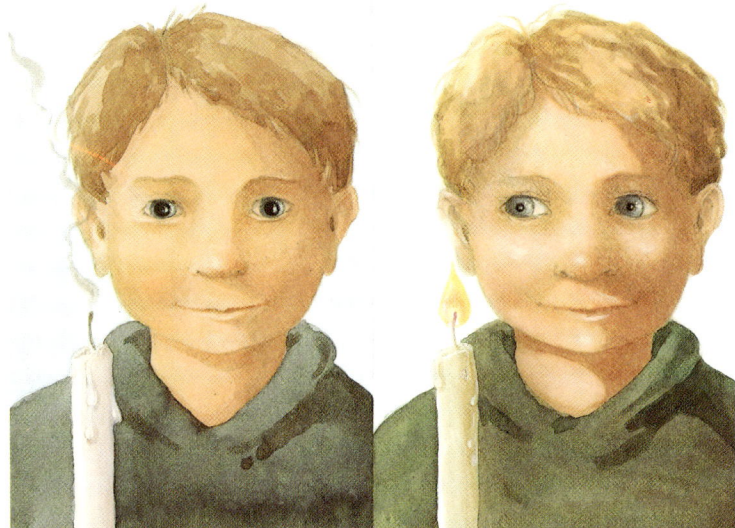

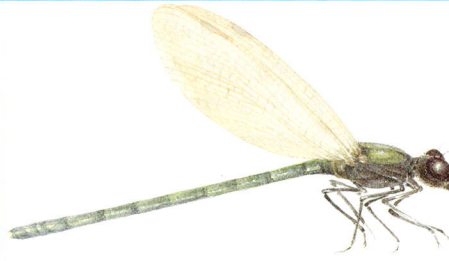

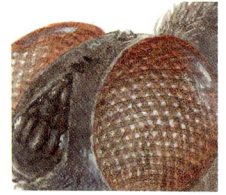

A short-sighted person sees distant things with a blurred outline. Glasses make the image clear.

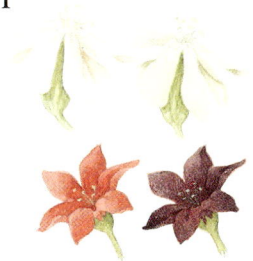

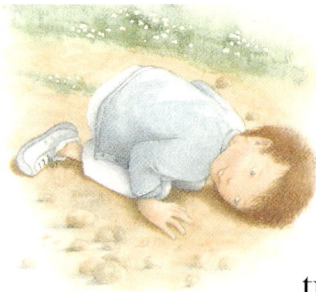

You can rest your eyes, but your ears go on working all the time.
They never stop picking up noises. Even in your mother's tummy, you began to know her voice. Later you learned to recognize different words, and then say them. From birth, your hearing worked as an alarm system, warning you of dangers before you could see them.

Outer ear
1. Auricle 2. Auditory canal

Middle ear
3. Tympanum (eardrum) 4. Ossicles (bones)

Inner ear
5. Semicircular canals
6. Cochlea

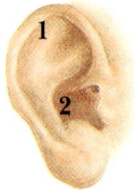

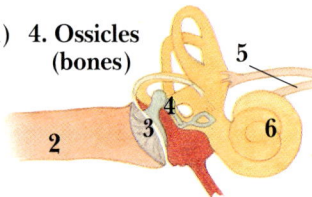

The tympanum is a very fine sheet of tissue which vibrates like a drumskin.
The louder the sound entering the ear, the more the tympanum vibrates. Behind it lie three tiny bones called the stirrup, the hammer and the anvil, because of their shapes. They transmit vibrations to the cochlea, a snail-shaped tube full of liquid. It turns the vibrations into nerve impulses which are sent along the auditory nerve to the brain. The brain works out where they come from and what they mean.

If you throw a pebble into the water, ripples move outwards from where it fell. In the same way, sound-waves move through the air.

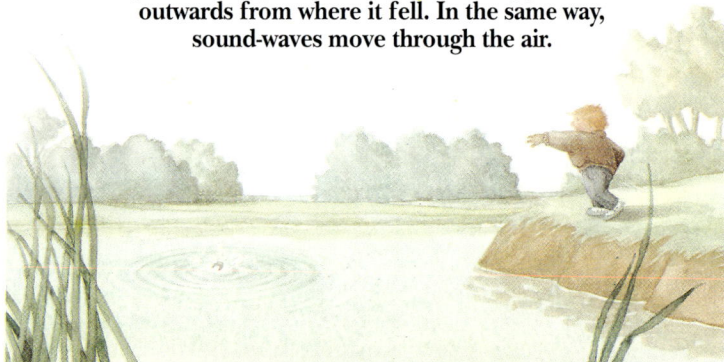

Try this experiment!
Stretch an elastic band between your finger and thumb. If you twang it, you will see it vibrate and hear a sound. Sounds are vibrations that move through the air.

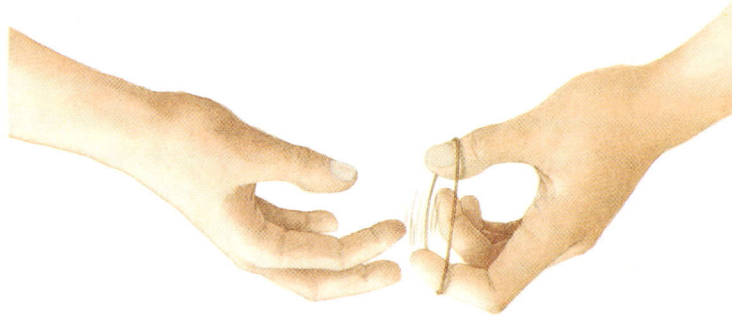

You can't hear every sound.
Ultrasounds are too high-pitched for us to hear, but a dog with its sharp ears will respond to an ultrasonic whistle.

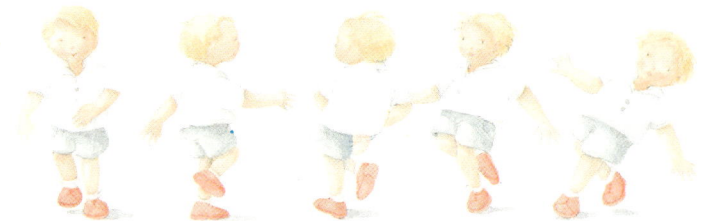

The semi-circular canals in your inner ear are the organs of you sense of balance.
If you spin round for a while, then stop, you will find it hard to keep your balance. This is because the liquid in your ears is still moving, even though you are not! The same thing happens when you feel sea-sick on board a boat.

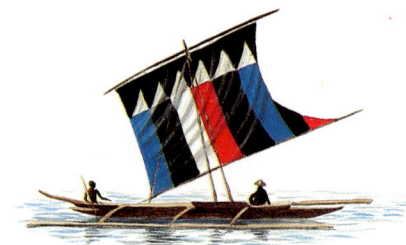

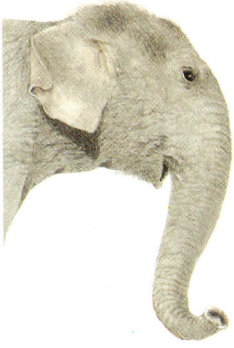

Crooked noses, long noses, squashed-up noses, turned-up noses... Noses come in all shapes and sizes, and the way they smell varies too. You could say a person's sense of smell is like their fingerprint: it is quite unique and different from anyone else.

What is a smell made of?

Countless tiny chemical particles float about in the air which you breathe. Inside your nose are smell detectors, called olfactory receptors, covered with tiny hairs. These receptors are bombarded with several thousand different smells.

Humans don't have a very acute sense of smell. Their receptors occupy a space of 5 square centimetres, whereas a cat's cover 20 square centimetres and a dog's may cover as much as 100 square centimetres. That's why sniffer dogs are used by the emergency services to find drugs, or injured people.

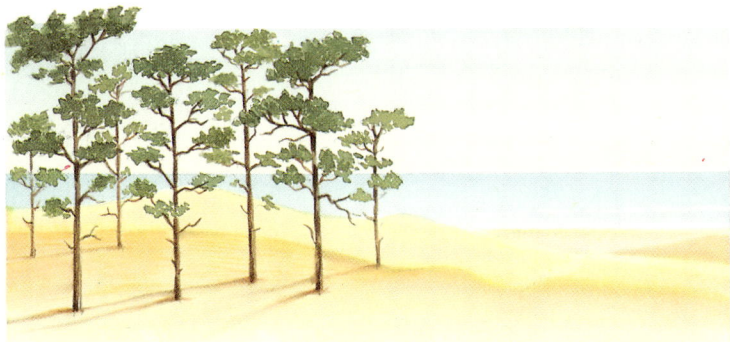

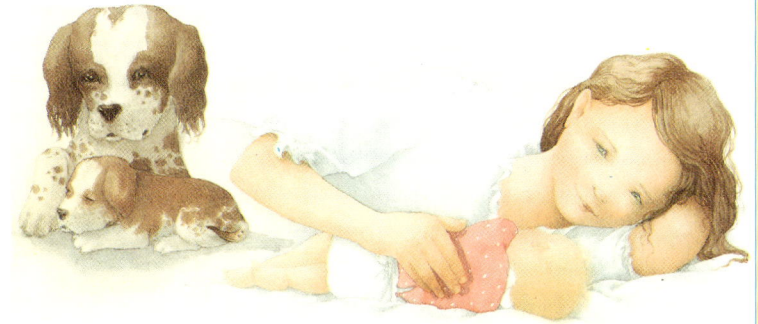

The receptors report the different smells to your brain, and your brain sorts out what they mean. A delicious smell of freshly baked bread wafting from the kitchen will make you feel hungry!

A newborn baby recognizes its mother's smell, and a mother can recognize the scent of her own baby.

This bond is very important. It comforts the baby and becomes the first means of communication it has with the world.

The scent linking mothers and babies is even more important among animals. Smell is often like an identity card. An ant colony will reject a strange ant passing by, because it does not smell right to them.

People who invent perfumes have a particularly well developed sense of smell.

They can detect the subtlest differences between scents and are able to pick out nearly four thousand different ones!

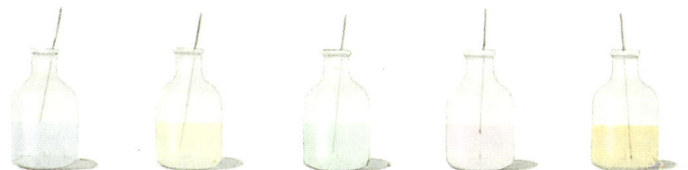

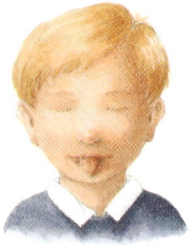

A child's taste buds are much more sensitive than a grown-up's.

Look at your tongue: it is covered with taste-buds.

They look like tiny spots, and aren't very pretty, but without them eating would be very boring indeed! Each one is sensitive to a particular kind of taste.

Our tongues are better at telling the difference between sweet and salt tastes than between bitter and sour ones.

Even before it is born, a baby prefers sweet-tasting things. Fortunately, the growing child learns to enjoy other tastes as well.

The tongue is sensitive to temperature and consistency, as well as to taste.

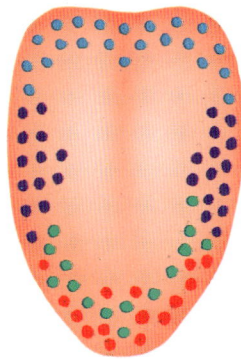

Keep your tastebuds exercised: try out different foods! Your sense of taste will improve as you learn to appreciate subtle differences in foods. You may even become a 'gourmet', that's a French word for someone who is an expert on food and wine!

- Bitter
- Salt
- Sour
- Sweet

The four basic tastes

are sweet (sugar), sour (lemon), bitter (chicory) and salty (salt).

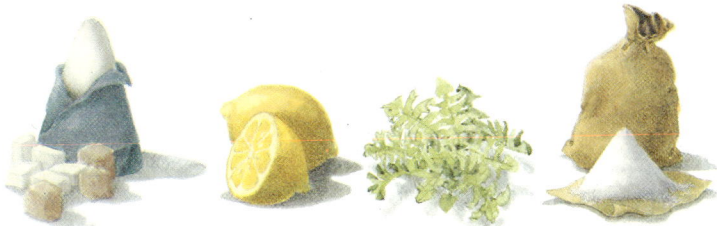

The sense of taste is closely linked to the sense of smell.

If you have a cold, it is difficult to tell what things taste like. The best way to take a horrible-tasting medicine is to hold your nose as you swallow it!

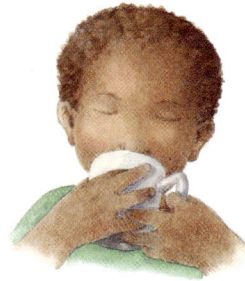

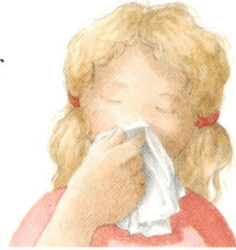

You may be left with a nasty taste in your mouth, but if the medicine is going to make you better, it's worth it!

Every country has different traditions about what tastes good: some peoples like very spicy foods, others prefer sweet ones.

French people like eating snails, wheareas many English people can't bear the thought of them! And how would you feel if you visited the Amazon and were offered a dish of grilled caterpillars, or roasted snake in Indonesia?

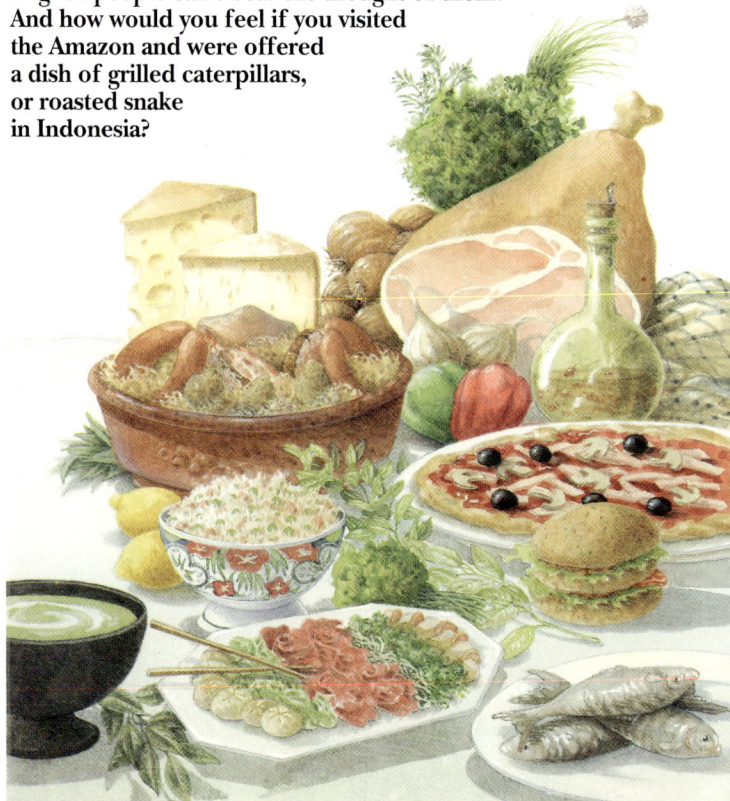

Your skin collects messages from the world around you.
It is sensitive to a gentle caress, the soft warmth of a jersey, the cold of an ice-cube, the prick of an injection.

Your skin reacts when it is touched.
Your skin is full of sensitive nerve endings. These can send messages in an instant to the zones of the brain which specialize in feeling. These then tell you how to react. For example, if someone treads on your toe, it hurts and your brain tells you to get your foot out of the way! Although it feels unpleasant, pain is very helpful: it's like an emergency siren warning us when something is wrong.

Some of the different impressions you feel when you touch.

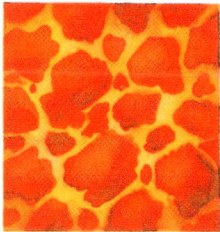 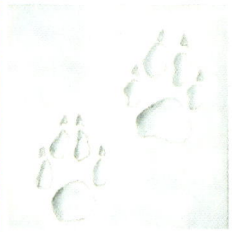 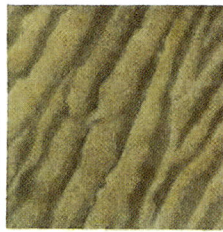

| hot | cold | rough |

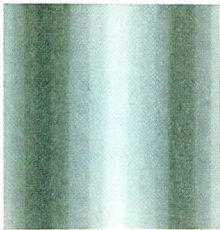  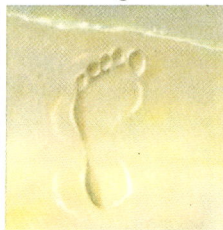

| smooth | soft | damp |

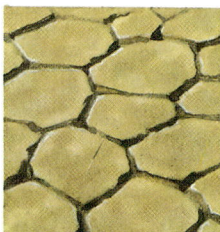 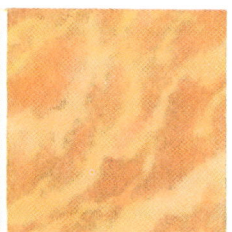 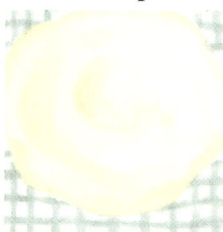

| dry | hard | wet |

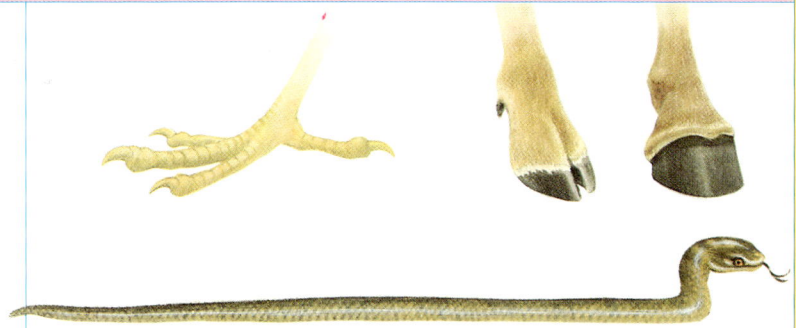

The scaly skin of a chicken's foot and the horny hooves of a deer or a horse are not as sensitive as the skin of a snake.

Babies explore the world around them by putting things in their mouths.
That is where the skin is most sensitive and they can learn a great deal. An injection is usually given on your arm or in your bottom, where the skin is less sensitive.

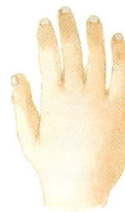 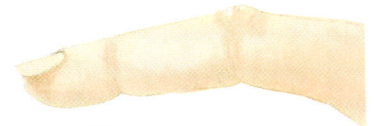

Our fingertips are very sensitive because we have a lot of nerve endings in them.

Animals have different ways of using their sense of touch.
What are they? Spiders are constantly spinning and then repairing their webs, using the hairs on their feet as their organs of touch. Bees can tell the shape of things very accurately by using their antennae. The tiny shrew uses its whiskers to find its way around its territory.

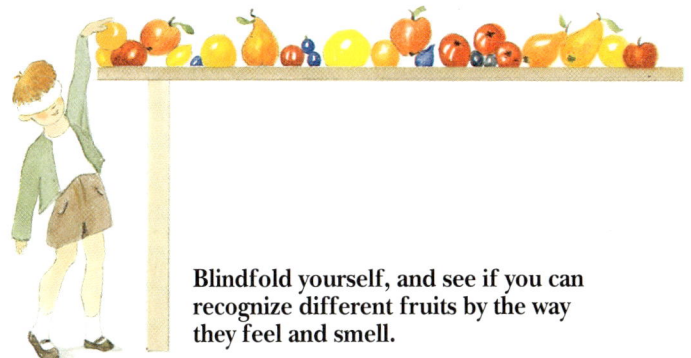

Blindfold yourself, and see if you can recognize different fruits by the way they feel and smell.

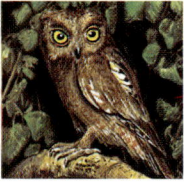

When the sun sinks down below the horizon, and its last pink rays fade from the trees and rooftops, you know that it will soon be dark and time for you to go to bed.
The birds begin to roost, cows in the field head for the byre, flowers close their petals and the family dog curls up in his favourite spot... But it's now that other creatures start to wake up! Owls, bats and badgers hunt at night, and sleep during the day instead. They are nocturnal.

<u>We spend about one third of our lives asleep.</u>
When you were a newborn baby, you slept nearly all the time, day and night. Now your life follows the pattern of the sun more closely, awake during the hours of daylight and asleep at night.

Early birds and night owls
Are you more awake in the morning or in the evening? People's body rhythms vary, and so does the amount of sleep each person wants and needs.

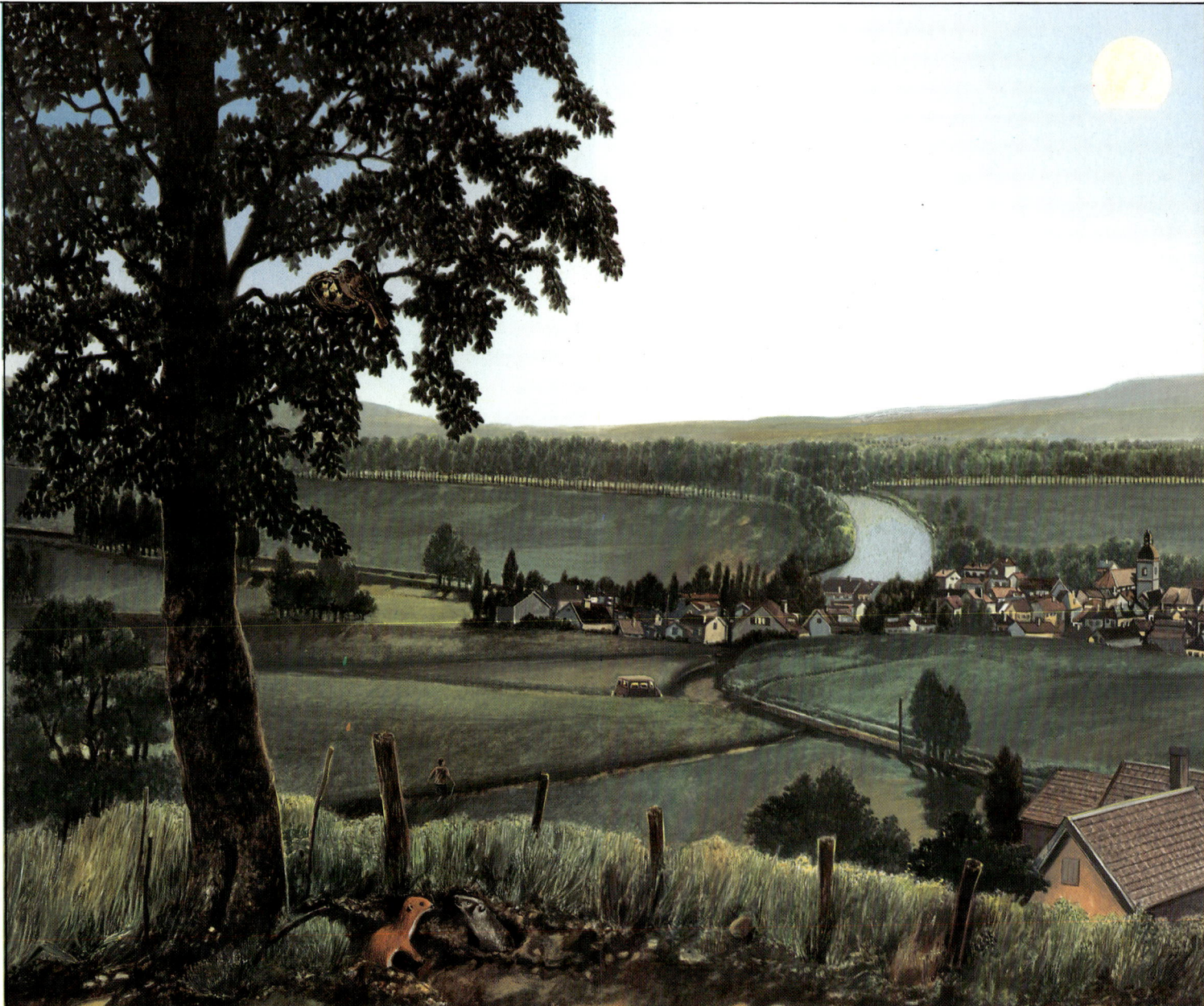

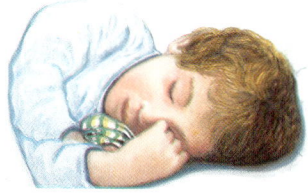

Children your age need a lot of sleep: at least ten or eleven hours each night.

How do you know when you're getting sleepy?
Your brain has been working hard all day. Now it sends signals that it's time to rest.

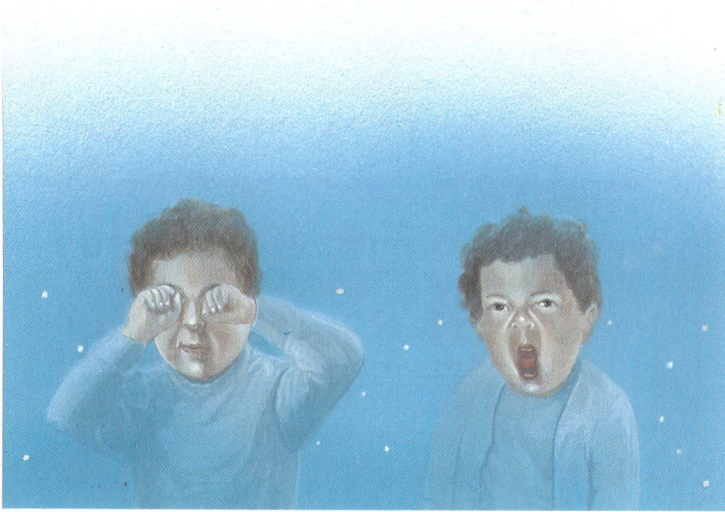

Your muscles relax, you start to yawn. You can't think straight and your eyelids feel heavy. Your eyes start to prickle, and grown-ups say, 'It's time for bed!' When you settle down to sleep, it helps to feel comfortable. Lie in your favourite position in bed, everyone has one that suits them best. Do you have a favourite toy that you like to cuddle?

Is it sometimes hard to get to sleep?
A drink of warm milk or orange flower water may help to send you to sleep. If you have a bath before you go to bed, it will warm you up and help you to relax.

Before you set off on this mysterious journey into sleep, ask someone you like to read you a story. It will help you feel happy and content.

It's important to feel safe. If you don't like the dark, leave the bedroom door ajar, or have a little nightlight burning. Once your body is quite at ease, relax your mind and think of lovely things... Goodnight, sleep well!

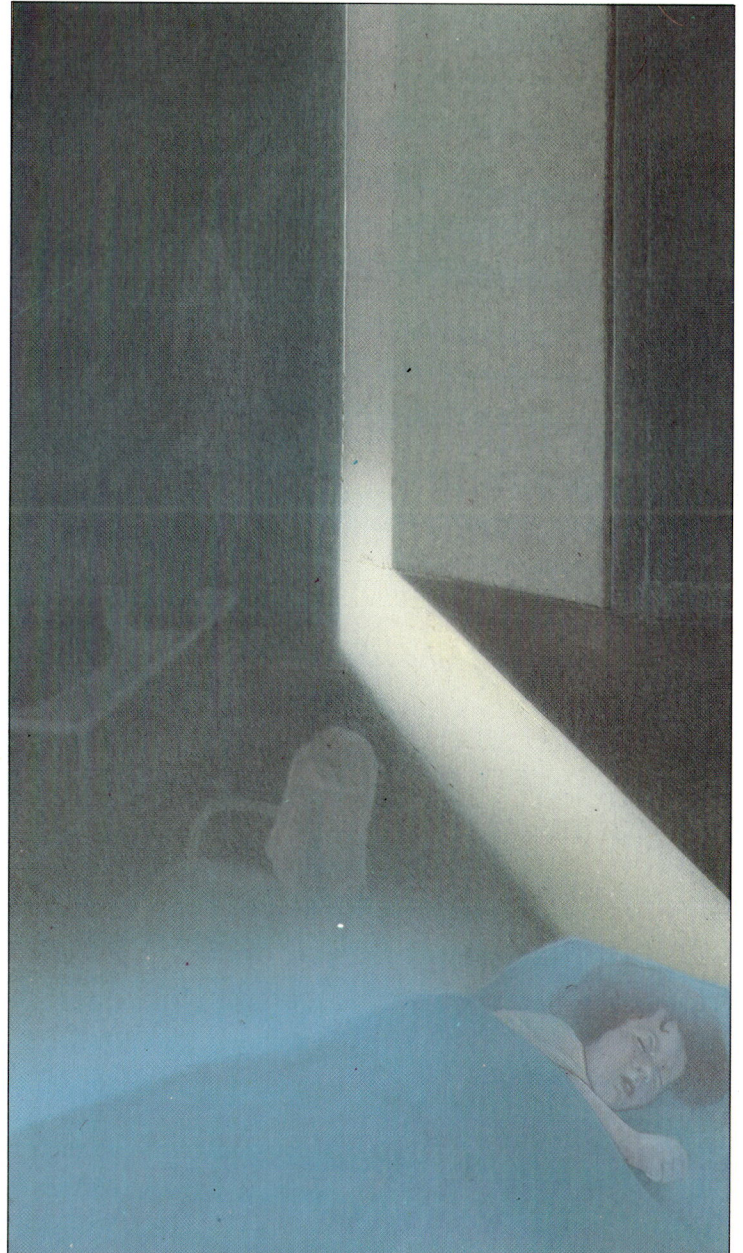

Each night, you go through several stages of sleep.

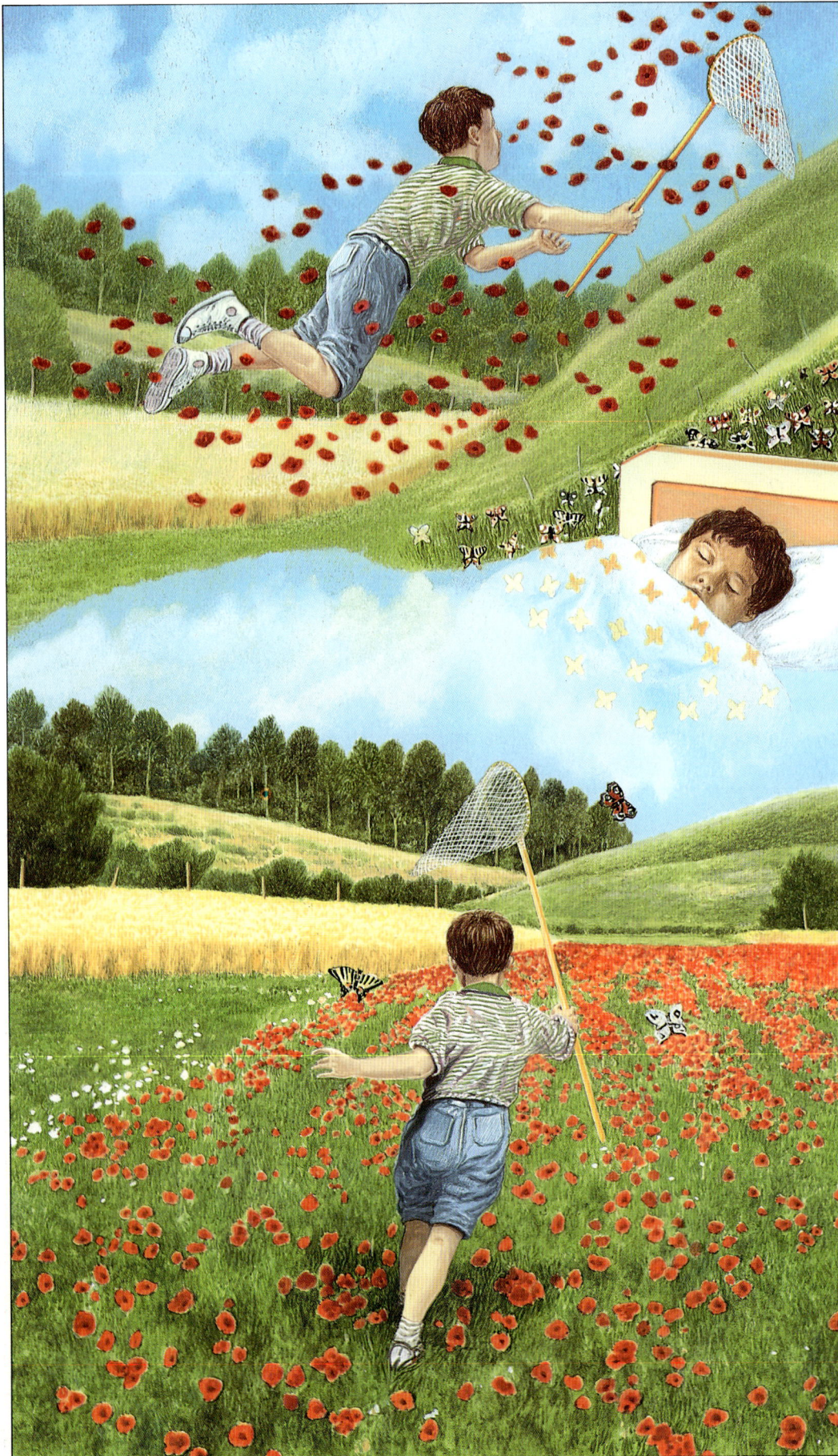

By measuring brain-waves, the electric signals given out by your brain, scientists have begun to find out about sleep.

It is made up of cycles: each lasts about two hours. You may go through four or five cycles in a night. Each cycle has several different stages.

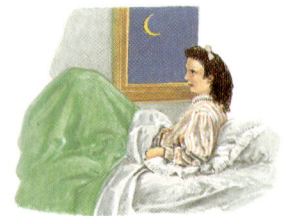

Insomnia is when you can't sleep.

At first you sleep lightly, then more deeply till you are 'sleeping like a log'! Then, under your closed eyelids, your eyes start to move rapidly about. You are deeply asleep, but the neurones in your brain are as active as when you were awake. You are dreaming.

In a period of deep sleep, you may snore or talk in your sleep. Some people even go sleepwalking.

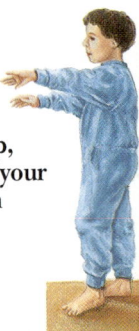

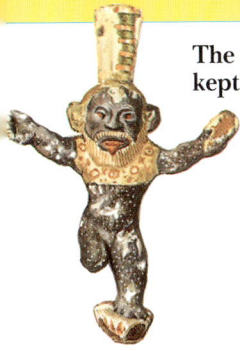

The ancient Egyptian spirit, Bes, kept watch over people as they slept.

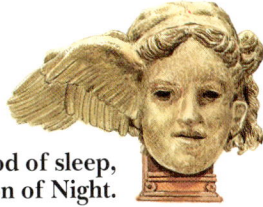

Hypnos, the Greek god of sleep, was the son of Night.

One cycle ends, another begins. When you have had enough sleep, you will wake up naturally at the end of a cycle. If your alarm clock goes off when you are in a deep sleep, it's a horrible shock – you feel as if you are coming back from a long way off!

Sleep is not a waste of time!

A lot of things happen when you're asleep, not just vital rest. Dreams help your brain sort out what has happened during the day; you grow, especially at the beginning of the night, as growth hormones are released. There's an old expression that 'sleep is a great healer'. You often find you wake up with the answer to a problem that was on your mind when you went to sleep. If you weren't allowed to sleep, you'd die. And if you weren't allowed to dream, you'd go mad!

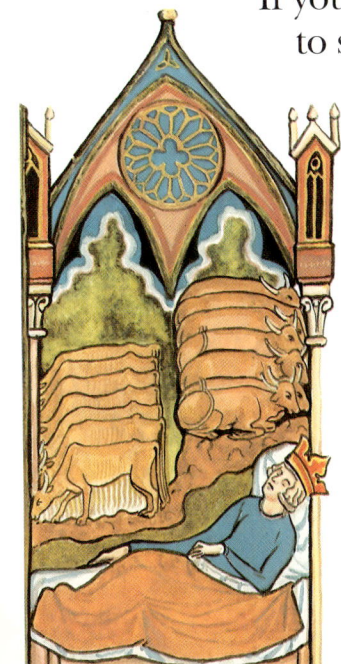

A Bible story describes the dream of an ancient Egyptian pharaoh: he dreamt that seven fat cows were eaten by seven thin ones. He was told this meant that Egypt would have seven very rich years, followed by seven years of drought and poverty. Apparently the dream came true.

Not all dreams are pleasant ones.

Sometimes you may dream of frightening things. You wake up with a jump, your heart racing. You need to calm down before you can go back to sleep again.

The meaning of dreams

During the 19th century, an Austrian doctor, Sigmund Freud, researched the meaning of dreams. He said that in our dreams our unconscious thoughts, all the things in our mind we keep hidden even from ourselves, come alive.

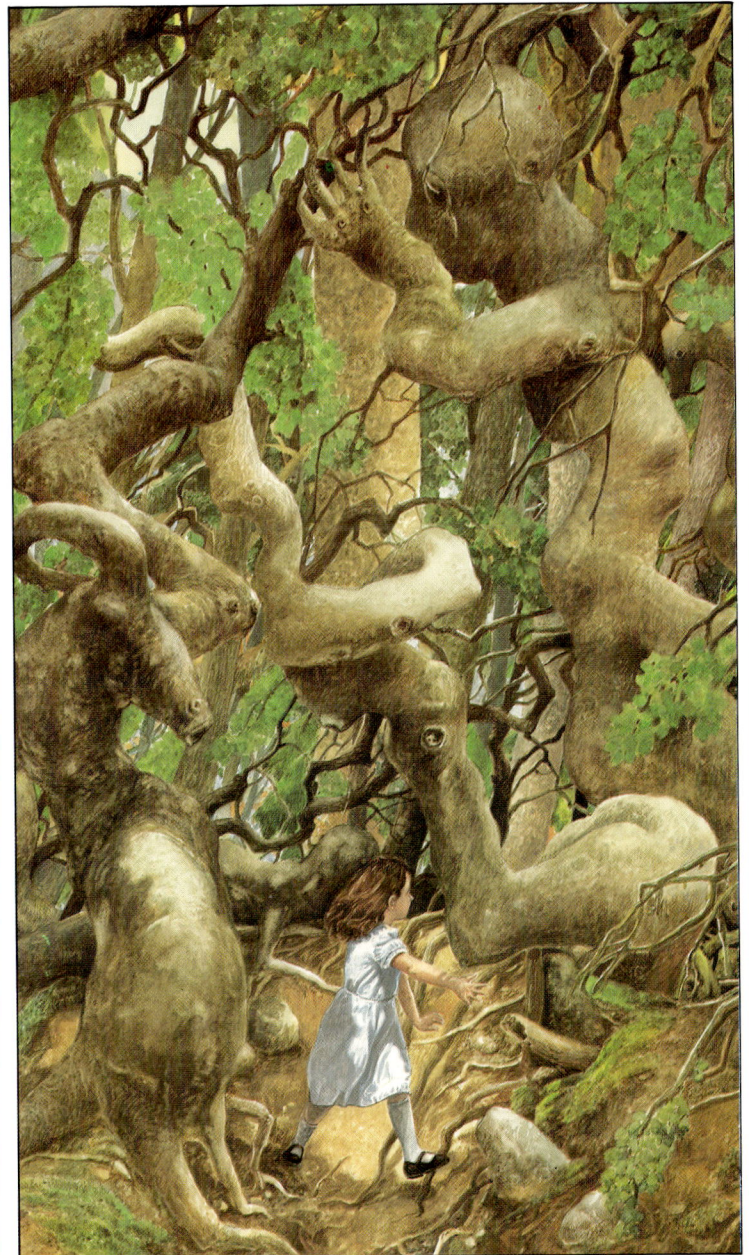

Germs are everywhere: in the air, in the ground, in our bodies.

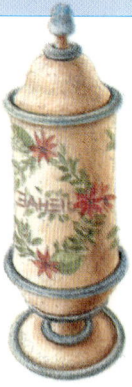

Have you ever heard anyone say, 'I've got a bug'? Germs are making them feel unwell.

What are germs? They are living things. There are millions of them, so tiny that you can only see them with a microscope. There are three types of germs: bacteria, viruses and fungi.

Bacteria are very small.
They develop and reproduce very fast by dividing into two. There are two types of bacteria: bacilli, shaped like little sticks, and cocci, which are round or oval.

Viruses are some of the smallest known living things.
They are not able to multiply on their own, so they live as parasites* inside living cells, which they destroy as they grow. If a virus gets into your body, you fall ill. The word virus means poison.

Fungi are microscopic.
One is called a fungus. They are often the cause of skin diseases.

Are germs ever useful?
Some bacteria are harmless. People have been making use of bacteria for hundreds of years, without realizing it.

Staying warm in bed is a good way to help your body to get better.

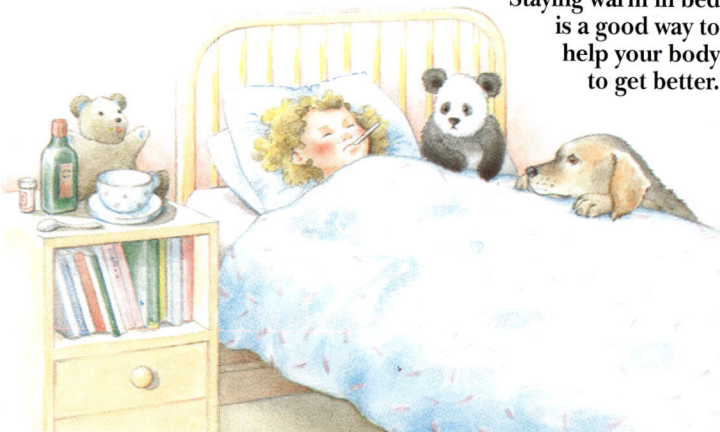

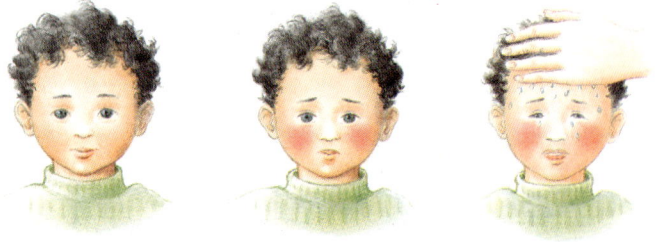

You're shivery and you don't feel well. You've got a temperature. These are all signs that you have an infection.

Bacteria make bread dough rise, and wine, beer and yoghurt ferment. Inside your intestines, there are billions of other bacteria which help your digestion. They are called intestinal flora.

Unfortunately, other germs are our enemies.
If they succeed in getting through your body's natural barriers – your skin, your tonsils and the hairs in your nose, the acid in your stomach – you may start to feel ill.

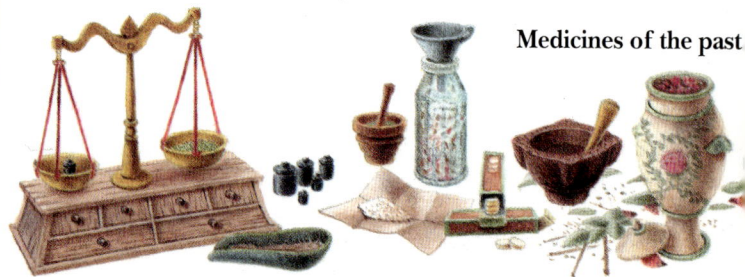

Medicines of the past

War breaks out between your body and the germ invaders!
Your temperature rises. This is one of your body's defence mechanisms, because heat kills off germs.

The lymph nodes in the lymph system near the infection swell up and harden, joining in the battle against infection.

White blood cells are like soldiers, sent into action to defend the body against the invaders. Your bone marrow speeds up production to make extra reinforcements.

Some bacteria are friendly, others are harmful.

Some illnesses are caused by bacteria.

Typhoid, cholera, whooping-cough, diphtheria, tuberculosis, tetanus, smallpox, leprosy, scarlet fever all used to be dreaded killer diseases that spread from person to person. Now, thanks to vaccinations* and antibiotics*, they can be controlled, and in most cases, cured.

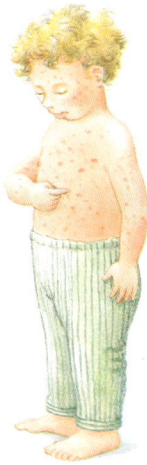

Some plants can be used as medicines... or poisons!

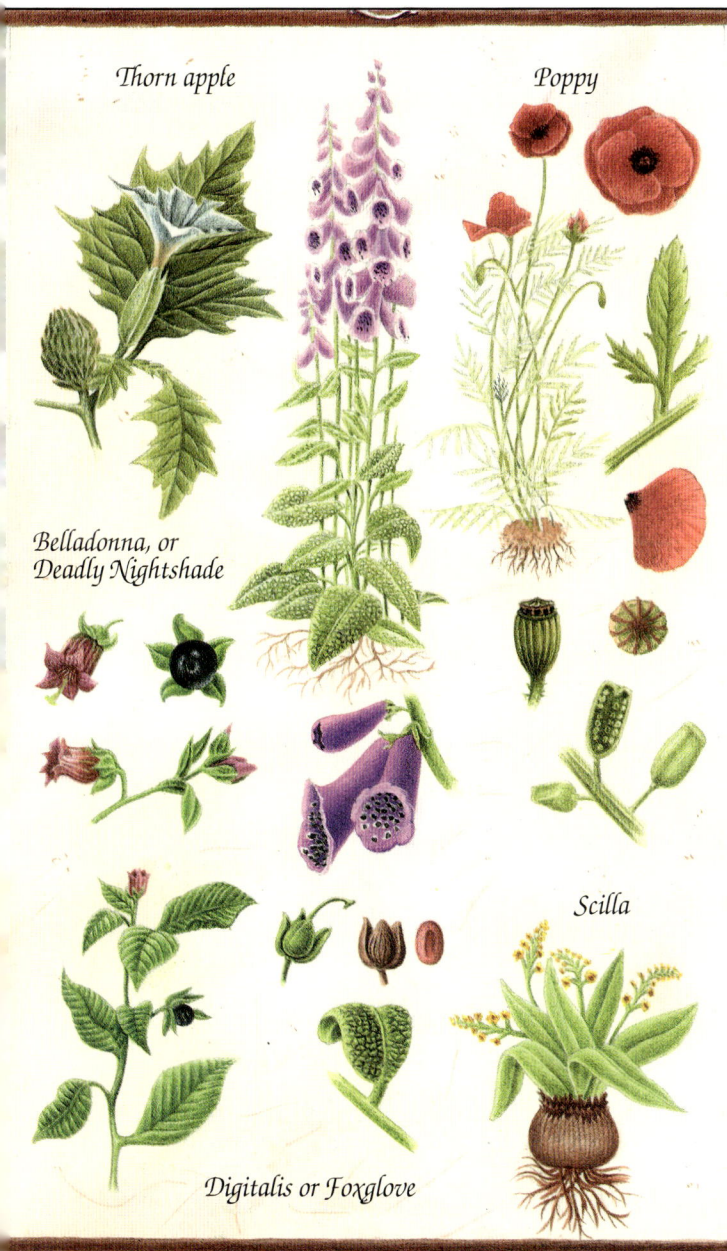

Thorn apple

Poppy

Belladonna, or Deadly Nightshade

Scilla

Digitalis or Foxglove

Some illnesses are caused by a virus.

Coughs, colds, sore throats, tummy upsets – these are often caused by viruses. So are most of the childhood illnesses, the ones you normally catch as a child. They are very infectious, and can spread like wild-fire through a class. Usually, you only get them once, because your body makes antibodies to defend itself. These stay with you for life, making you immune to the disease. Measles, chicken-pox, german measles and mumps are all caused by viruses, and are rarely very serious. Certain types of 'flu (influenza), and yellow fever, hepatitis and poliomyelitis are more dangerous. Many illnesses caused by viruses can be avoided, thanks to vaccinations.

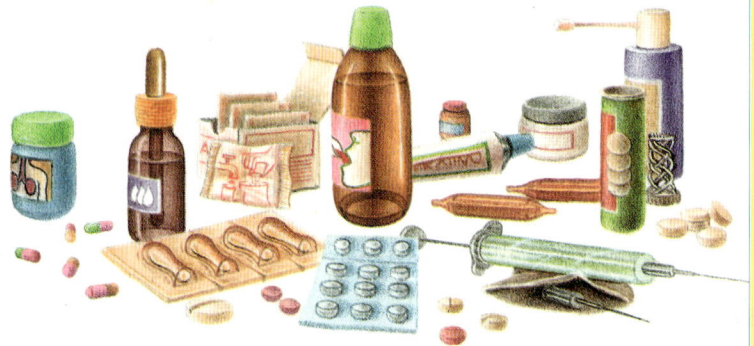

How do we take medicines? As pills or syrups, as drops or ointment applied directly to the infected area, as suppositories to push up inside our bodies, or by injection.

Cancer: an illness that is not caused by germs

Abnormal cells in one part of the body can start to multiply and group together to form a lump, called a tumour. No-one knows why they start to behave like this, and unfortunately it is a difficult process to stop. If the tumour or lump is malignant (harmful), cells from it may break away and damage other healthy cells, spreading the disease. Often it is possible to destroy the tumour or reduce its size.

Louis Pasteur: the pioneer of vaccination

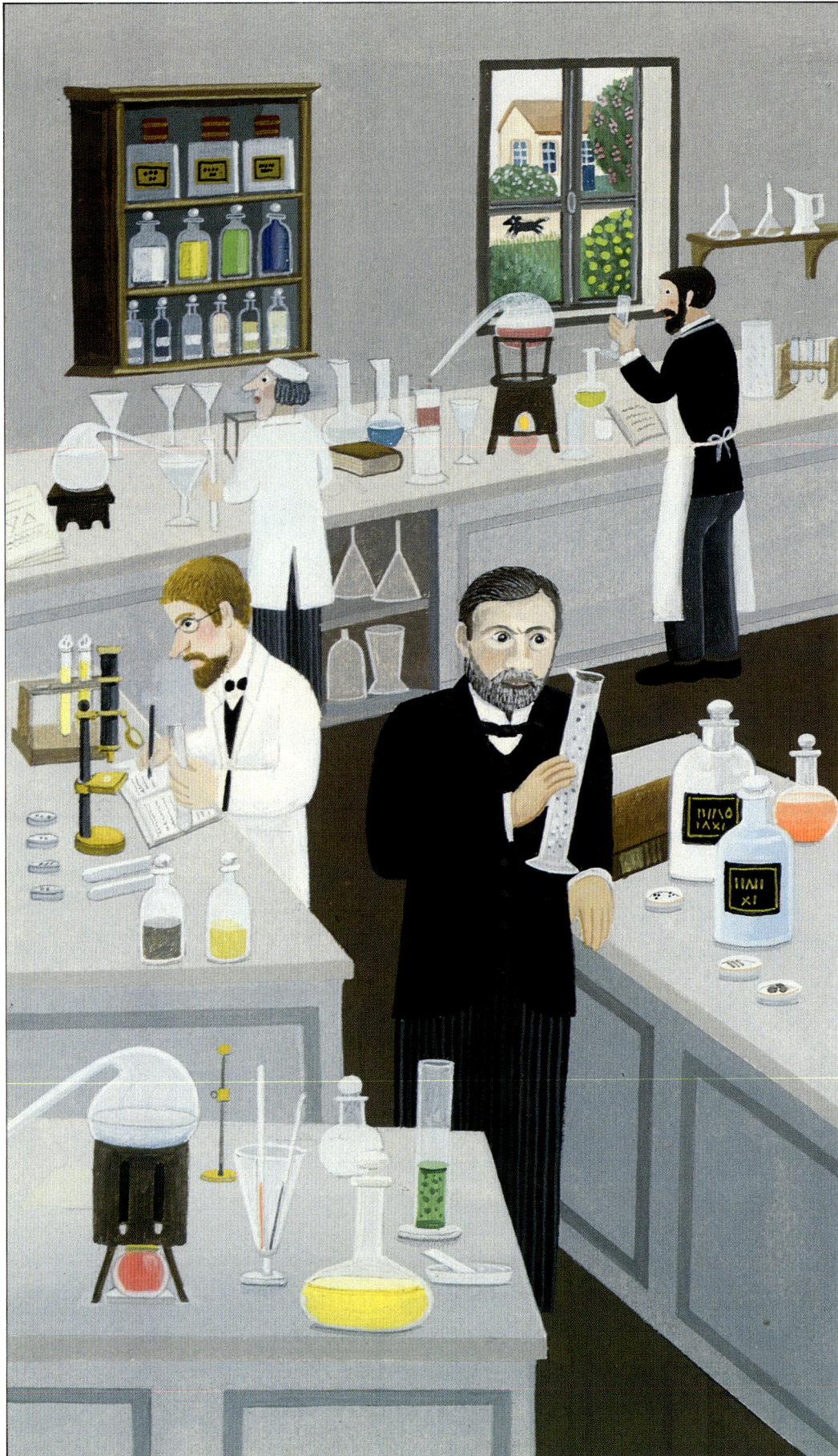

During the 19th century, a French scientist called Louis Pasteur discovered that it was possible to destroy harmful bacteria in milk if it was heated to a very high temperature. This 'pasteurized' milk would keep for several days.

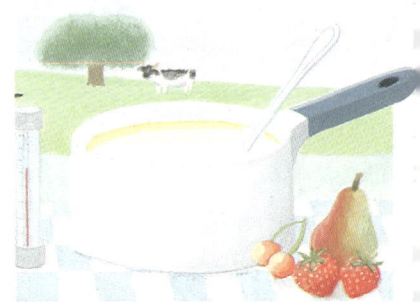

The discovery of vaccine
Now that he knew how to weaken bacteria, he became interested in human illnesses. He discovered that if he injected his patients with a dose of weakened bacteria, they did not seem to get worse; in fact, the germs seemed to strengthen the body's natural defences. Pasteur had discovered the principle of vaccination, and saved his first patient, a boy who had been bitten by a rabid dog, from the deadly disease of rabies in 1885.

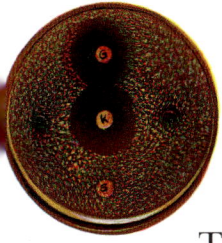

Viruses are more difficult to kill than bacteria.

No medicine, no antibiotic can kill a virus. It's not very easy to get rid of them! The only way is to teach the body to defend itself on its own. An important part of your body's defence system are the antibodies made by the white blood cells. They destroy harmful bacteria and viruses, and neutralize the poisons they produce. Sometimes a particular germ may prove too strong, but if the antibodies win, they remain in the body to destroy that germ if it should ever reappear.

Vaccinations give you protection in advance.

When you are vaccinated, you are injected with a very weak dose of a certain virus. Your body starts to produce a stock of antibodies against it. If you come into contact with the same virus again, it will not make you ill. Babies are more at risk from illness before they have been vaccinated.

Making a vaccine

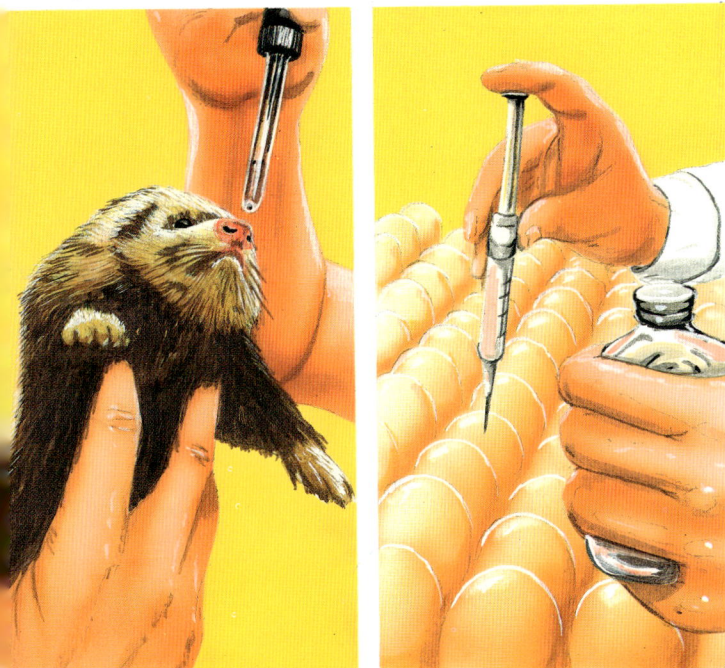

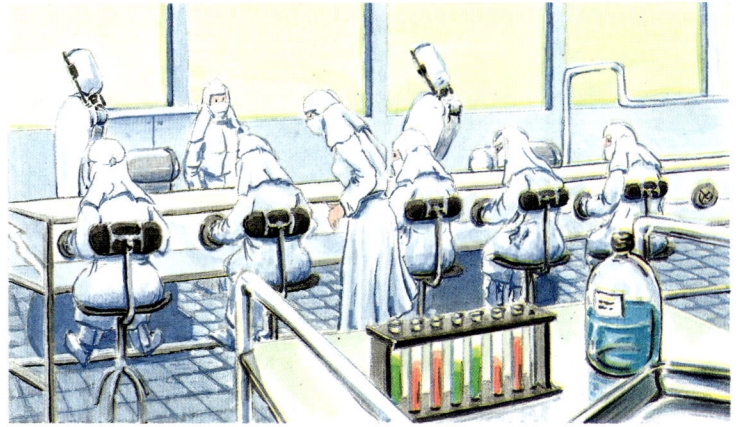

A research laboratory

The older you get, the more germs you meet, and the stronger your defences grow.

New vaccines are discovered through research.

Since Louis Pasteur, many more vaccines have been discovered to deal with tuberculosis, diphtheria, tetanus and many of the illnesses caused by bacteria which used to be fatal. Now you can be vaccinated against all childhood illnesses except chicken-pox. Sometimes, even if you have been vaccinated against them, you can catch mumps or measles, but only in a mild form.

The trouble is, new viruses keep appearing! Doctors first recognized the AIDS virus in 1980. We now know a lot about the virus, but in spite of a huge amount of scientific research, no-one has yet found a vaccine against it. It is a deadly illness, which attacks the body's defence systems. A person who is suffering from AIDS is unable to fight off infections and, sadly, eventually dies.

To make a vaccine, the virus has to be grown, or 'cultivated', on living animal matter: here, fertilized eggs are being used in the manufacture of 'flu vaccine.

If you are seriously ill or you need an operation...

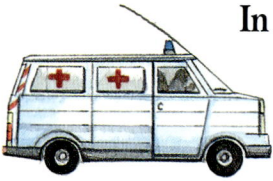
Ambulance

In hospitals, nurses and doctors work in shifts to give you care 24 hours a day. If there is an emergency, no time is wasted: all the equipment is there on the spot, and doctors specializing in certain illnesses, or different parts of the body, can be at your side within minutes.

Samples of blood or urine, which may help in diagnosing* an illness, can be sent down to the hospital laboratory immediately. An operating theatre can be made available in case of an emergency. X-rays and body scanners using very clever equipment can show doctors pictures of the inside of the body.

Everything in an operating theatre is kept as clean as possible to avoid infection. Doctors and nurses wear hats, masks, gloves and gowns, and cover the patient with drapes.

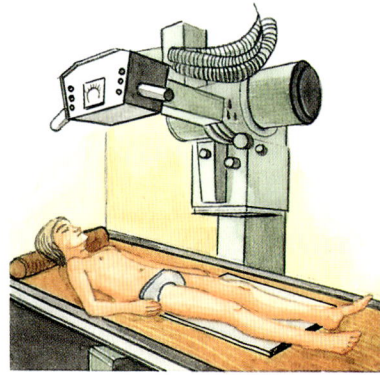
Radiography: an X-ray is being taken.

What if the surgeon decides to operate?

Don't worry! The doctors will explain what's going to happen. You are wheeled to the anaesthetic* room, where the anaesthetist gives you an injection. You have a lovely floating feeling, and you're asleep before you know it. When you wake up, the operation is over. You can hardly believe it: you think you're still waiting to go into theatre!

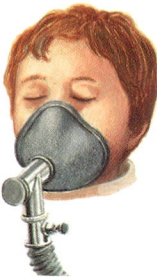
Sometimes the anaesthetist gives you gas to send you to sleep.

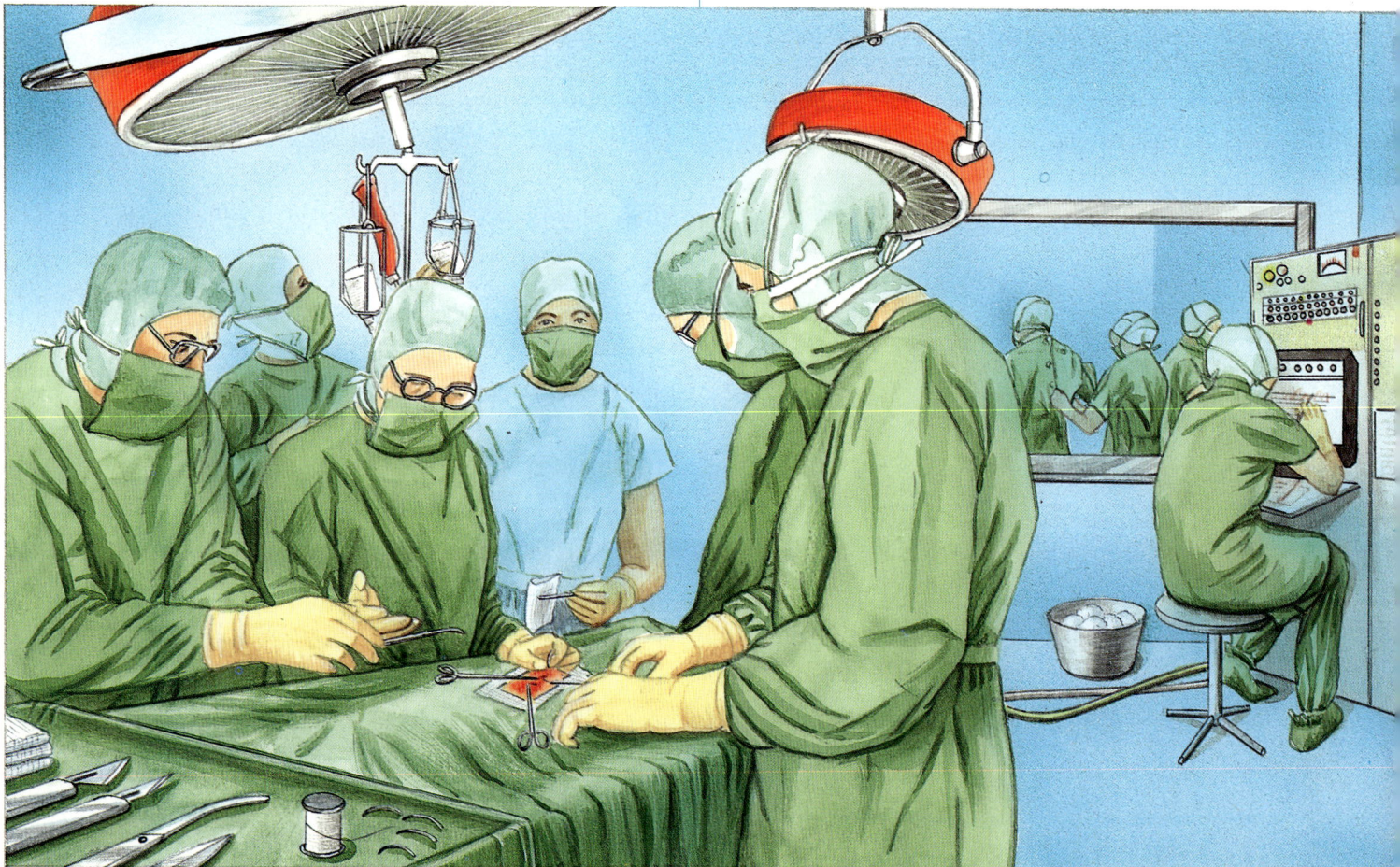

A day in hospital

You get better quickly in hospital. You stay in a big room where all the other patients are children too: it's called a paediatric ward. It's very comforting to see that you aren't the only one who is ill, and often you make very good friends.

The mornings are kept for medical tests and a visit from your doctor.

You may be surprised to find that hospital isn't very restful! You are woken up early, because the mornings are busy: there are examinations to carry out, you may need an X-ray... If you are too ill to walk, you may be taken to the X-ray department in a wheelchair. Your doctor comes to see how you are in the morning, too.

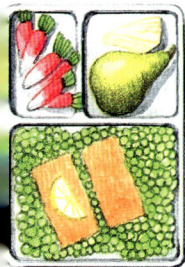

In the afternoon, your friends and family can come and visit you.

Lunch is early in hospital. There is always a choice, and usually the food is good. Afterwards, there's time to rest before your visitors arrive.

Then you can play in the games room, or watch television. Children who have to stay in hospital for a long time have lessons as well – just when you thought you had escaped school!

It's not always very easy to get to sleep at night, because hospitals can be noisy places. But it's reassuring to know there is always someone looking after you. You'll have a lot to tell your friends about your stay in hospital when you go home.

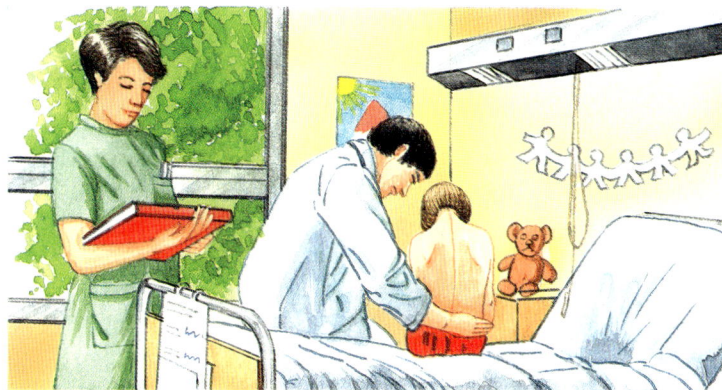

Your doctor comes to see you on his ward round.

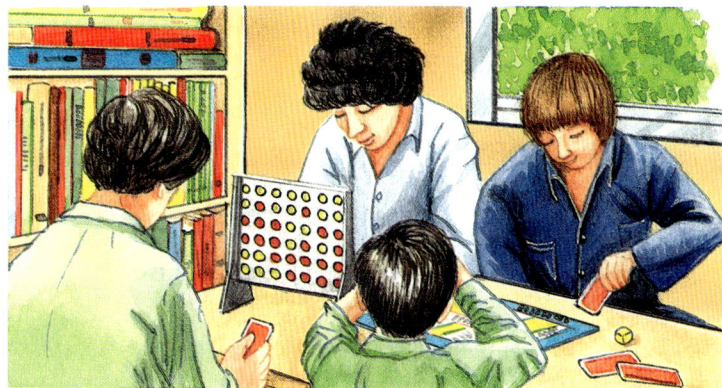

Young patients can go and play in the games room.

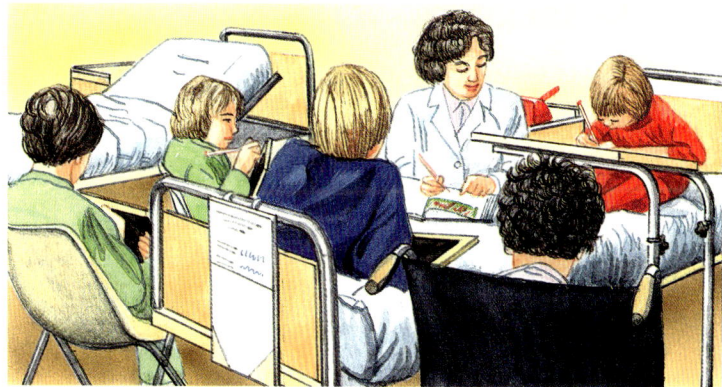

Teachers come and give lessons to children who have to stay in hospital for a long time.

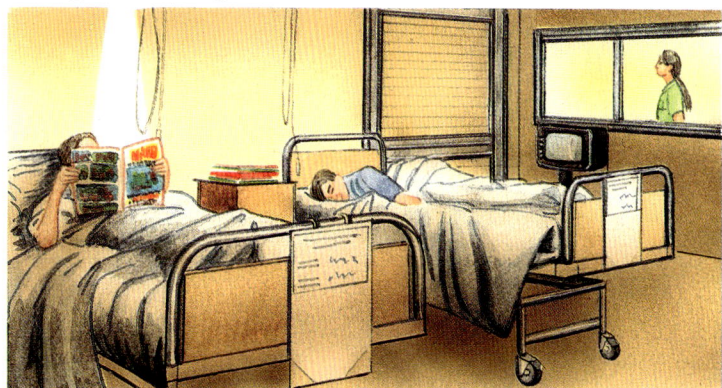

At night, there are always nurses on duty in the ward.

Your body is like a well-designed machine.

A very clever machine which runs beautifully, but you must take care of it!

From time to time, the machine breaks down, sometimes seriously, and you have to repair it. Modern medicine has made so much progress that doctors can now put right a lot of the things that go wrong. One of the best ways to prevent the germ invaders taking hold is to keep your body as healthy as possible: eat well, take plenty of exercise, keep yourself clean and give yourself enough sleep.

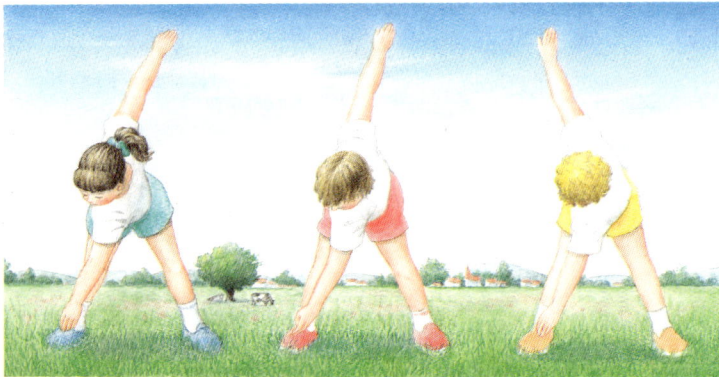

There is nothing like doing a sport that you enjoy. Physical exercise is vital for a healthy body.

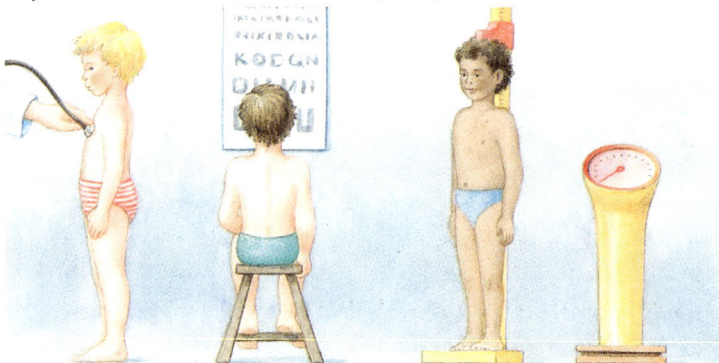

At a child health clinic, your height, weight, sight and hearing can be checked, and vaccinations given.

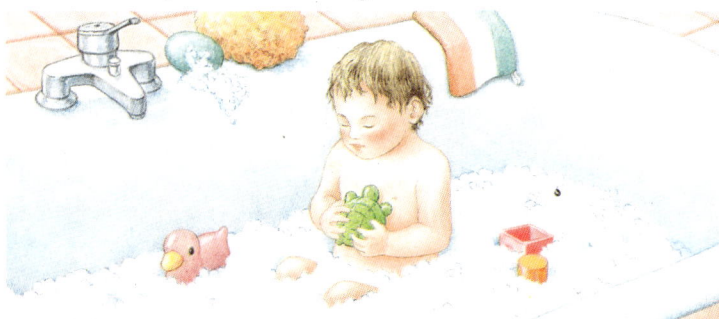

You ought to have a good wash every day. You'll rub away the old layer of sebum, and a new one can grow in its place.

It's good to stretch yourself, to try to improve, to exercise your mind and body... Pick something you like doing, be realistic about your capabilities, and do it at your own speed. Sometimes, before you try, you may not feel like making an effort, but afterwards there's such a sense of achievement!

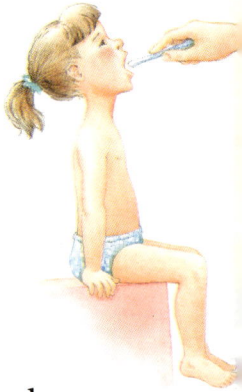

A healthy mind in a healthy body

Everything cannot always go according to plan, but that should not stop us having confidence in ourselves. We are all different each one totally unique and special. Did you know that the people who live longest are those who keep alert and active? It's never too late to learn something new!

Personal hygiene is very important.

Always wash your hands after you've been to the lavatory, to clean off any germs. Don't forget a daily wash all over! Soap cleans germs off your skin, and toothpaste gets rid of germs round your teeth. A scratch or graze may need a little disinfectant ointment.

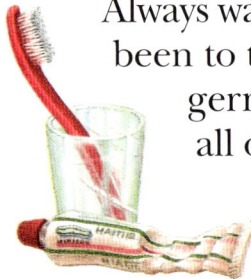

Your body needs exercise!

Keep fit by being active, playing sport regularly and enjoying the fresh air outdoors. The machine must be kept running or it will start to rust up!

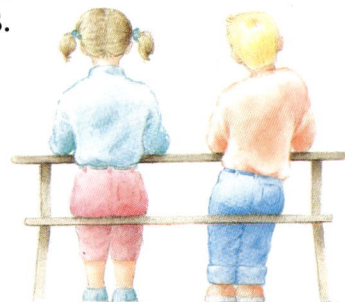

Try always to have good posture.

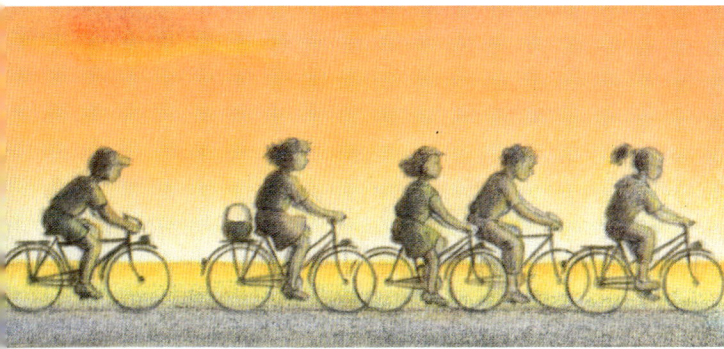

Eat all sorts of different foods!

Not too much, not too little, but a variety every day! A good breakfast is a good start to the day. Your body needs a boost of energy after several hours without food. One of the great tragedies of our time is that, in certain parts of the world, thousands of people die of malnutrition every year. Weakened by lack of proper food, their bodies aren't strong enough to fight off disease and infection.

Make sure you have enough sleep.

You must give your body time to rest if it is to grow up healthy and strong. Don't go to bed too late: an hour's sleep before midnight is worth two afterwards!

Regular check-ups

Like an engine, your body needs a check-up from time to time. Your doctor will make sure all is well.

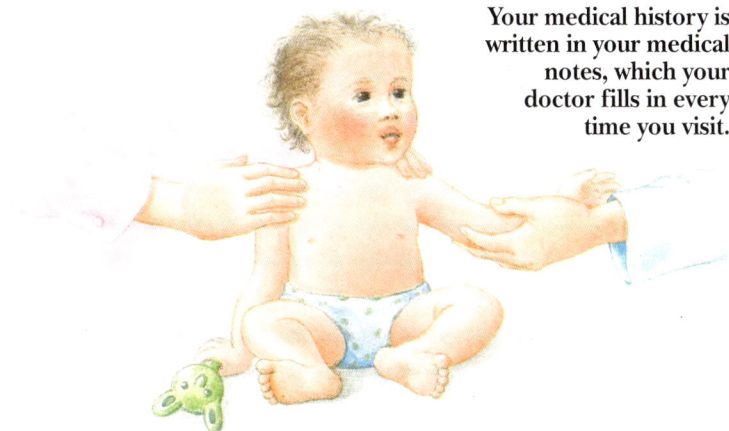

Your medical history is written in your medical notes, which your doctor fills in every time you visit.

Babies grow and change so quickly that they need to be seen by a Health Visitor* or doctor at least once a month. They should have a series of vaccinations between about 12 weeks and 6 months. Older children need boosters, to keep the vaccinations up to date. A dentist should check your teeth at least twice a year.

All the medical checks in the world are not enough, though, if you don't try to know your own body and look after your health!

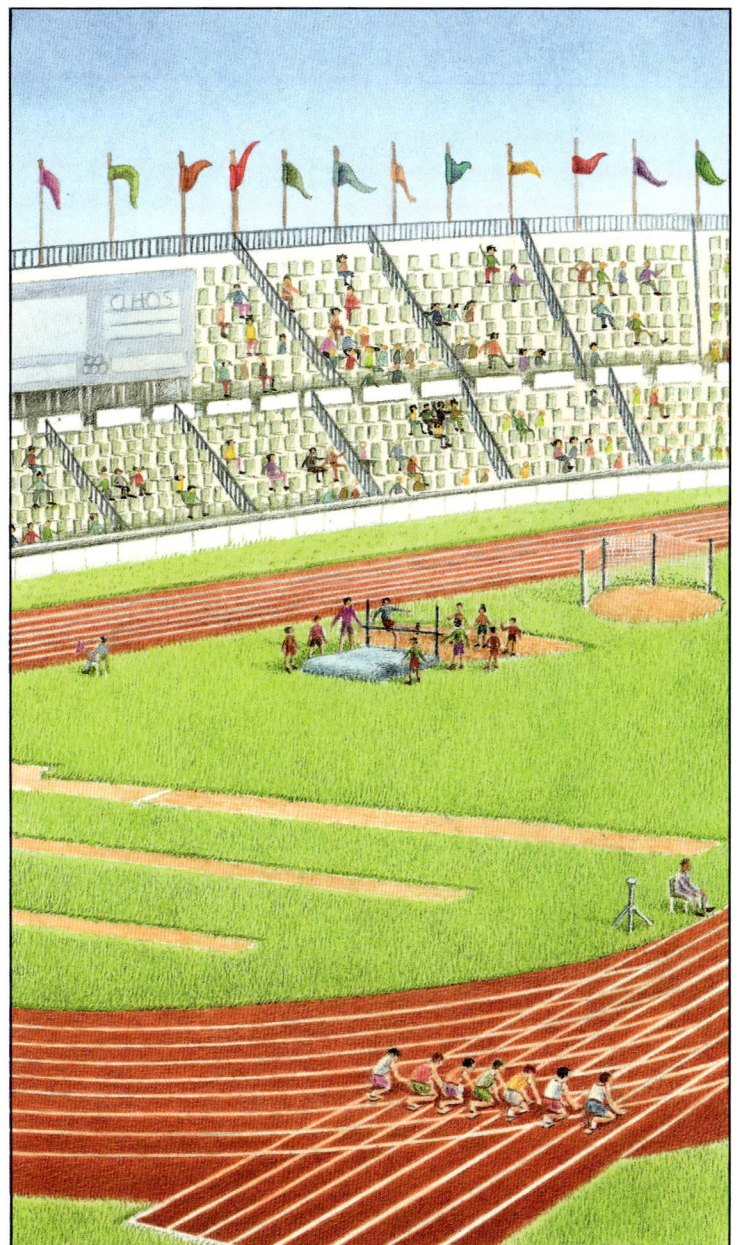

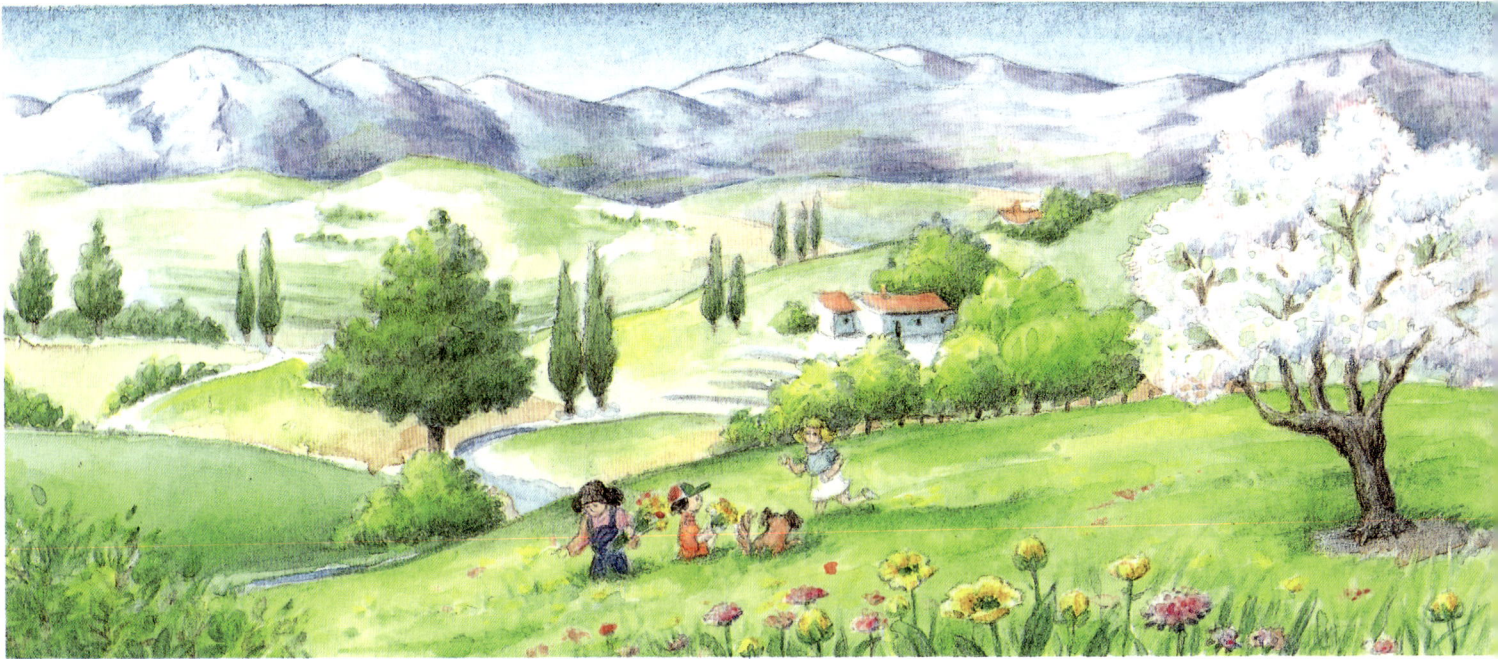

The rhythms of life

Each person's body has a built-in rhythm, which follows the course of day and night, and the seasons, warm or cold. Some people are more active in the evening, and like to get up late. Others are early birds and prefer to go to bed early too. There are people who have to work all night long, like nurses and shift workers in factories. Their internal clocks have to adjust to different rhythms.

Animals and plants have their rhythms too.

A cat can sleep just as well during the day as at night. Many animals in the wild are constantly on guard against their enemies, and only get snatches of sleep: giraffes don't sleep for more than ten minutes at a time! But monkeys and birds may sleep for twelve hours or more.

The life of a plant follows the rhythm of light and dark. Daisies, tulips and water-lilies keep their petals shut until daybreak.

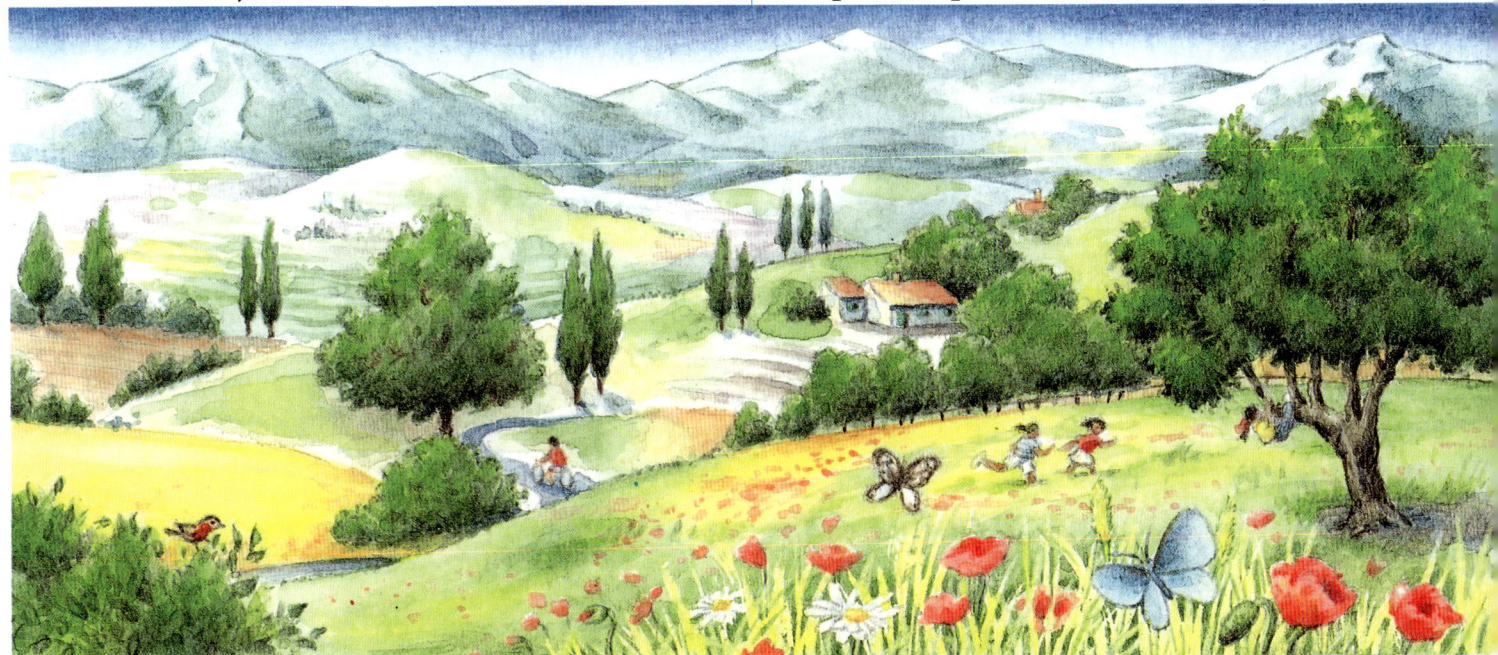

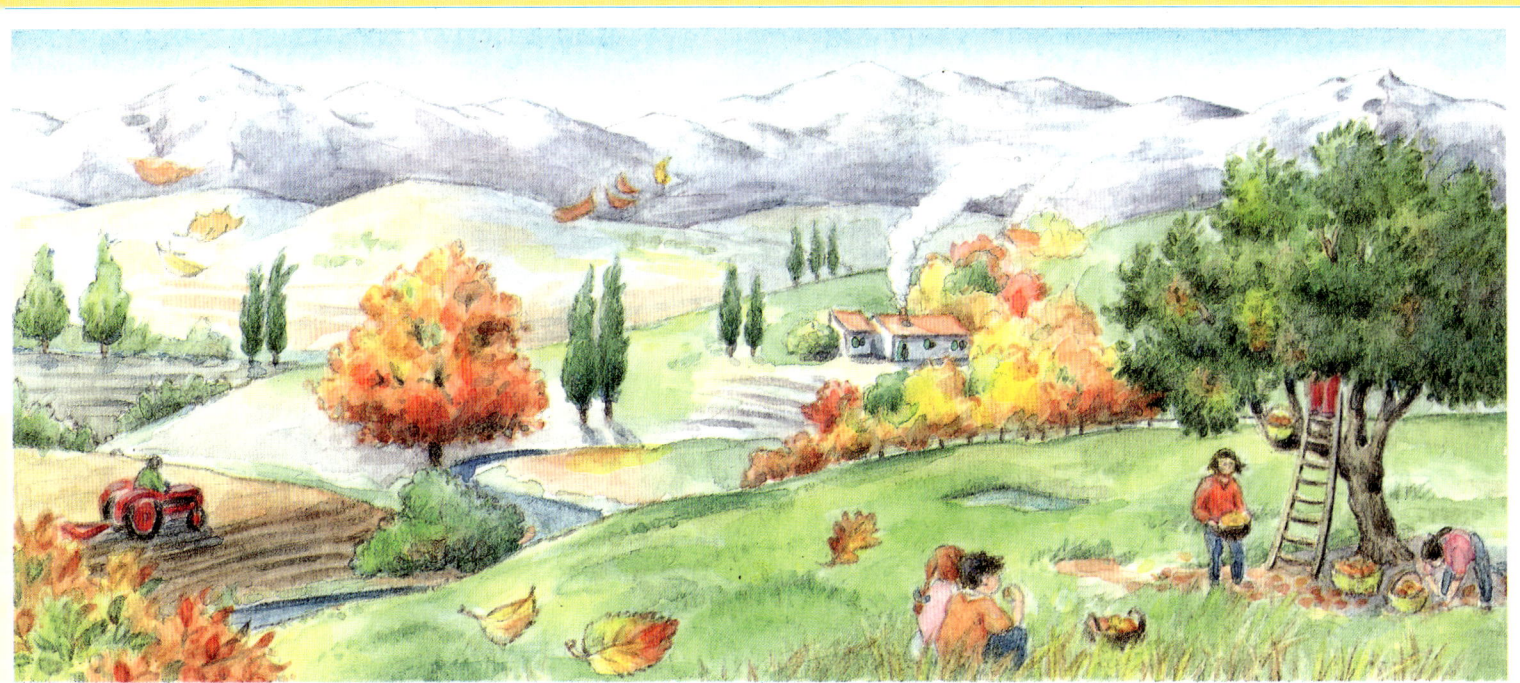

Everyone has a built-in clock.

It regulates how our bodies work. At night, though, we don't simply switch off: many things go on as we sleep. Large amounts of growth hormone are produced, to help repair or replace damaged tissue. Our body temperature is lower in the morning: it rises with all the activities of the day. When you travel abroad to a different time zone, it takes a few days for your internal clock to catch up with your watch.

Following the rhythms of the seasons

Some animals spend the winter asleep. You might like to as well – it's hard to get up on those cold, dark mornings! In the spring, the warmer weather lifts your spirits and seems to give you new energy. The summer sunshine tops up your body's supply of Vitamin D, which you will need to help you through the winter. In autumn, nature slows down. But it's back to school for you, perhaps with a new teacher and a new class.

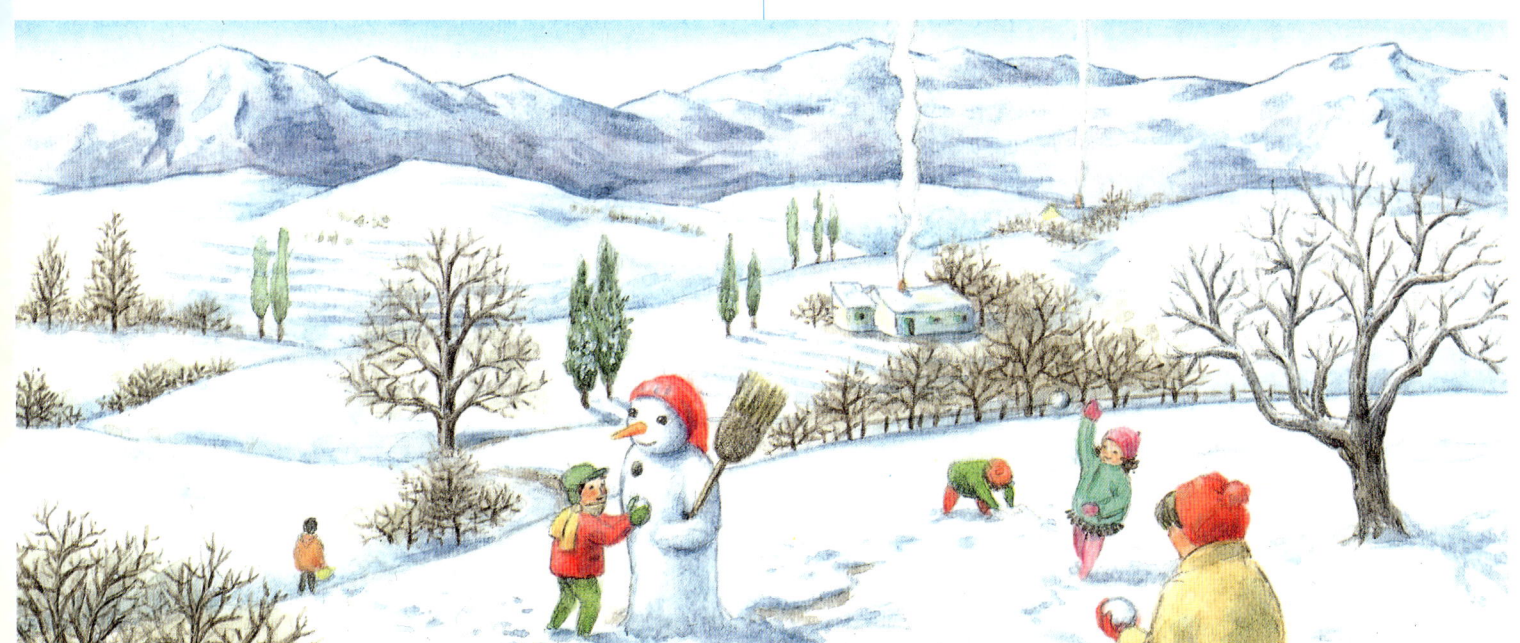

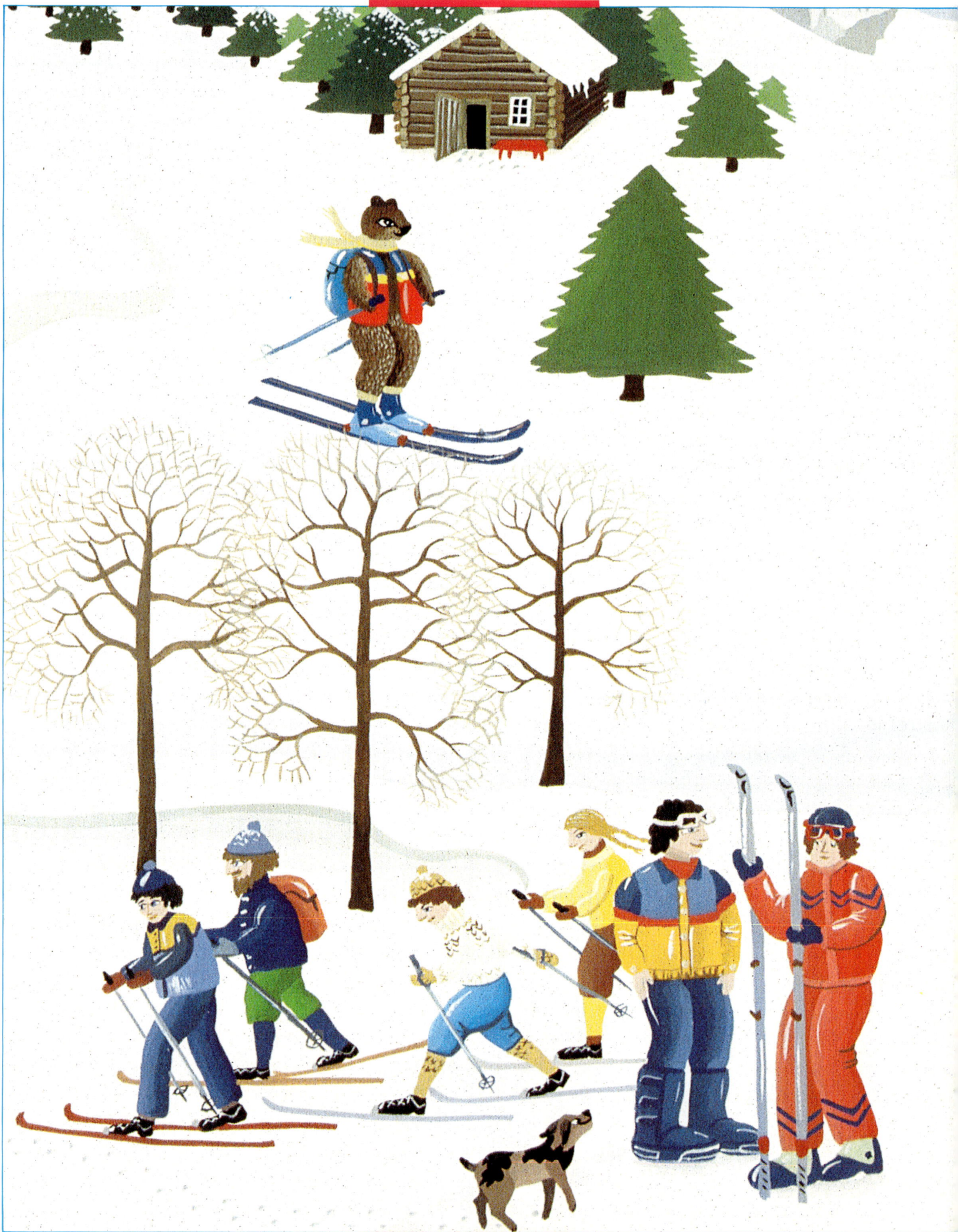

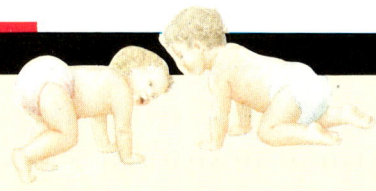

Games and activities, a quiz, intriguing facts, a glossary, followed by the index

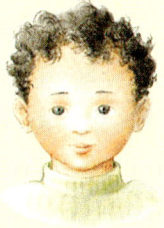

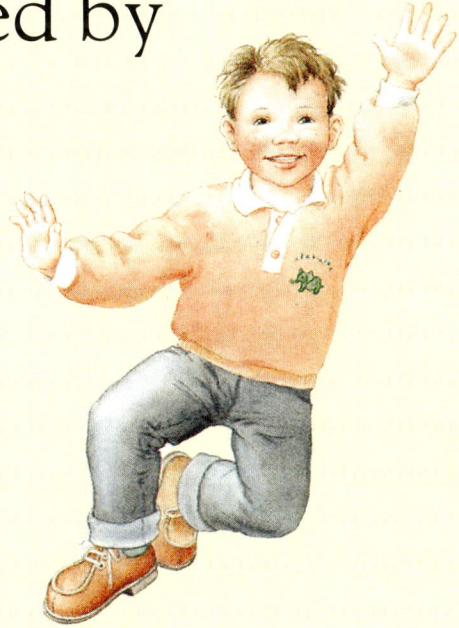

Different ways to celebrate a baby's birth.
In certain countries, special bread is baked, beautifully decorated to look like a little baby. Sometimes the loaf is made in the shape of the placenta, as a reminder of how the baby was fed until it was born.

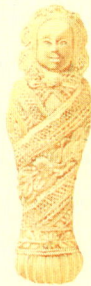

In some parts of Africa,
the placenta is buried in the ground, and a tree is planted over it. The tree will belong to the child, who can watch it grow as he or she grows, from year to year.

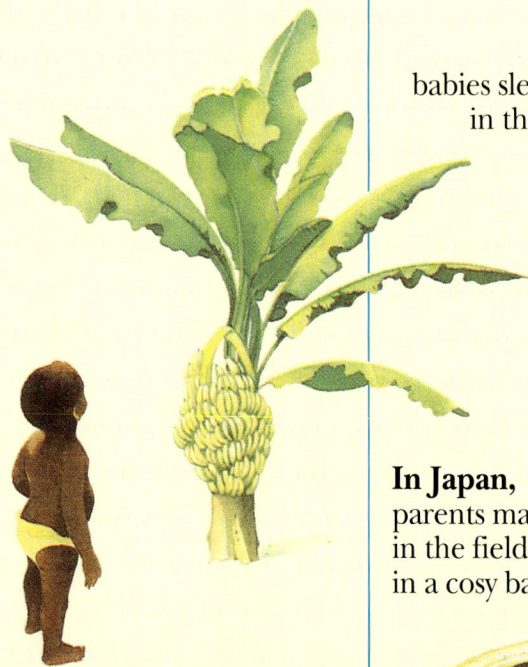

In hot countries, babies and children don't need to wear very many clothes.

There are all sorts of places where a baby can sleep!

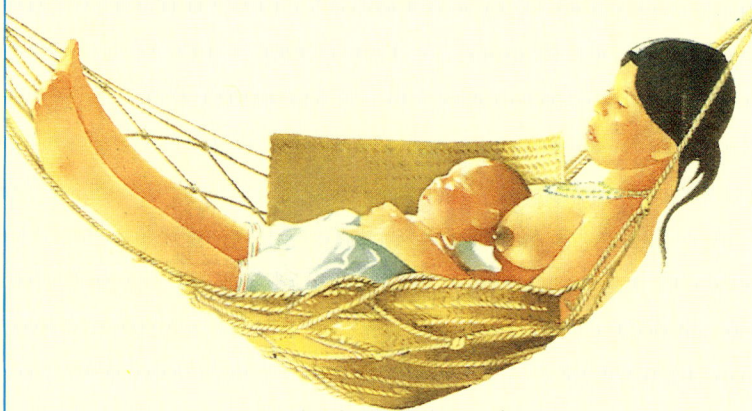

Amazonian Indians in South America
put their babies in hammocks, and they sleep hanging above the ground. They are safely out of the way of any crawling insect which might give them a nasty bite.

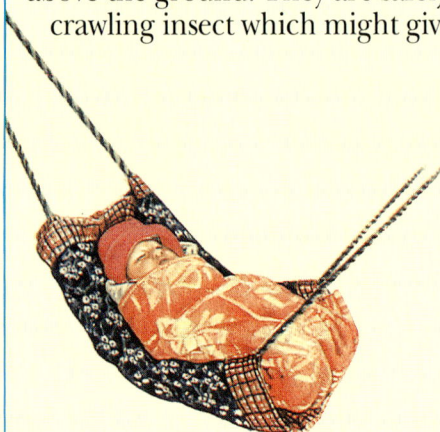

This Chinese baby is sleeping soundly in a sort of hammock made of cloth.

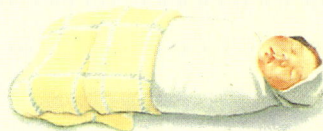

In Mongolia,
babies sleep on the carpet in the big family tent.

Western babies
often sleep in cots which rock or swing, just as they did long ago.

In Japan,
parents may take their babies to work in the fields with them, tucked up in a cosy basket like this.

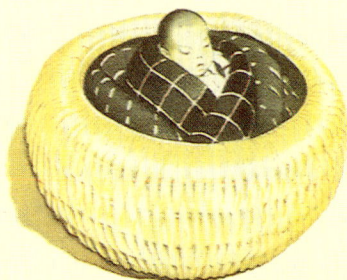

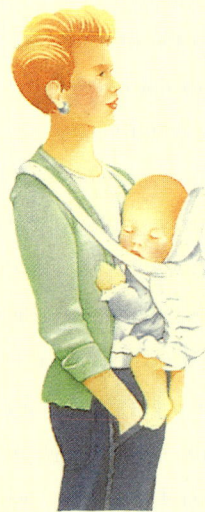

Babies long ago
Babies used to be wrapped up snugly in wide bandages called swaddling bands. If a mother could not feed her baby, she would hire a 'wet-nurse' who would breast-feed that baby as well as her own.

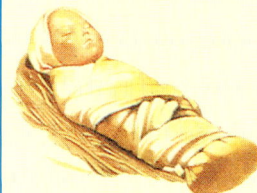

A new-born baby in the 12th century

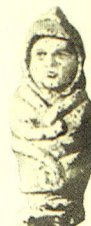

Roman baby

The first bottles
for babies were invented in the 18th century. They were horns filled with cows' milk.

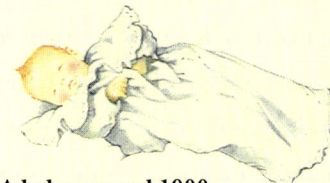

A baby around 1900

About 1850, babies began to be dressed in long, wide dresses so that they could kick their legs.

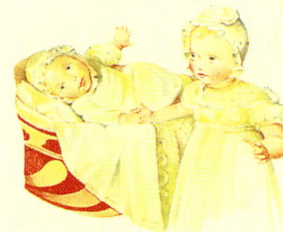

Nowadays,
babies can be as active as they like. They are very soon dressed like the rest of the family.

■ Did you know?

In the Middle Ages, few people had a proper bed. The whole family slept on the same mattress, which was made of straw or leaves.

Up until the 18th century, children slept in their parents' bed. Later they shared a bed with their brothers and sisters.

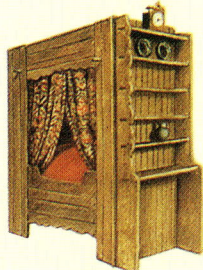

A country-style box bed

Towards the middle of the 18th century, houses began to be built with a new room: the bedroom, separate from the living rooms. Beds became narrower.

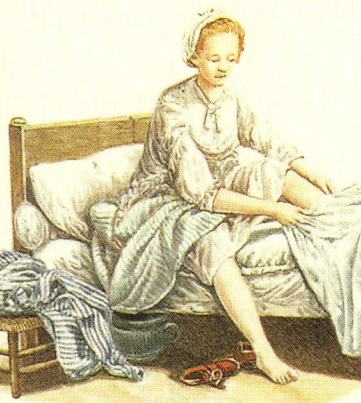

It's less than one hundred years since children have slept one to a bed, and more recently still that they have been given a room of their own.

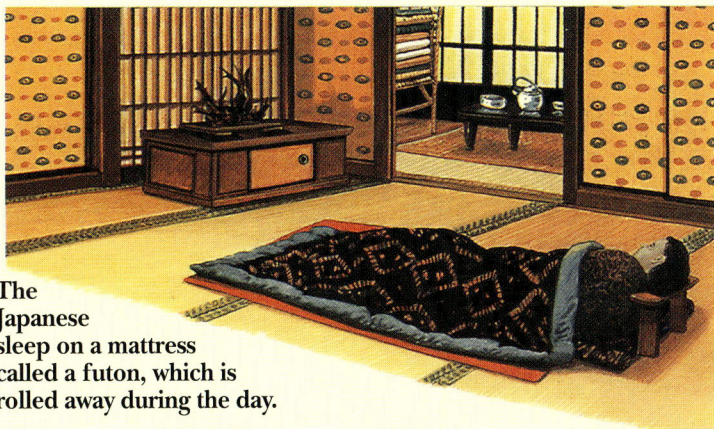

The Japanese sleep on a mattress called a futon, which is rolled away during the day.

Every country has its own customs. There are lots of different ways to go to bed.

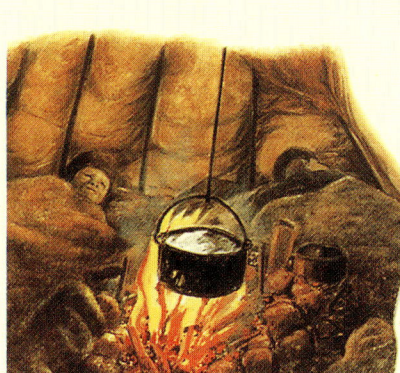

Lapplanders sleep on a mattress of branches, covered with reindeer hide.

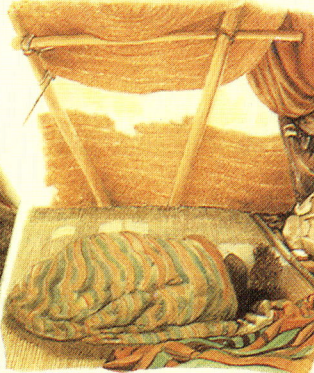

In Morocco, some people sleep wrapped in a blanket on the carpet of their tent.

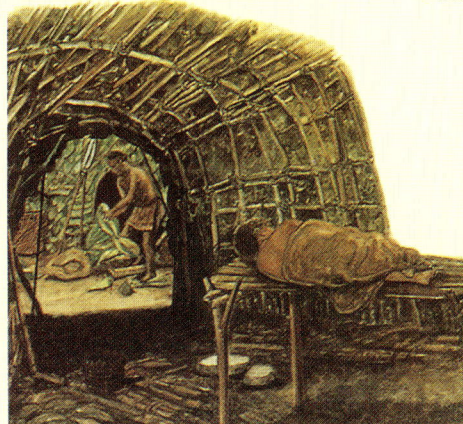

Pygmies lay out sleeping mats on a sort of platform, safely above the creepy crawlies on the ground!

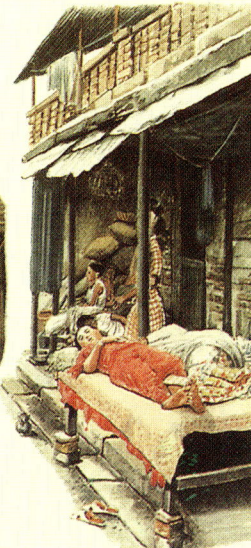

In India, people sometimes bring their beds out onto the pavement when it's hot.

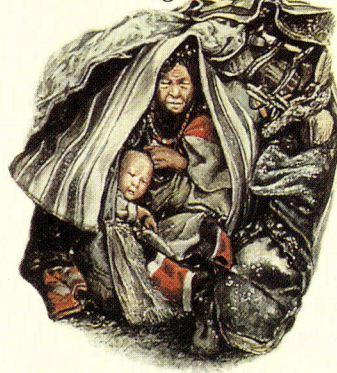

When they are on the move, Tibetans go to sleep simply wrapped up in blankets.

Beds from the past
Long ago, beds used to be highly decorated.

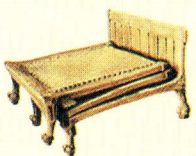

An Egyptian bed

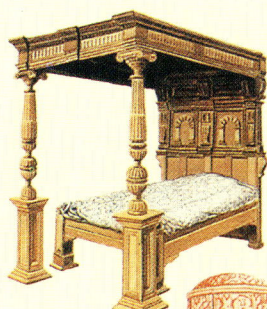

A four-poster bed in the classical style

Polish bed, 18th century

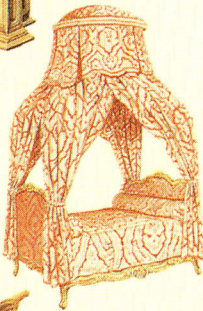

Raised, boat-shaped bed, of the 1800s

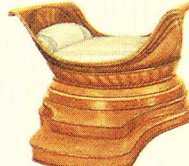

Bed of State

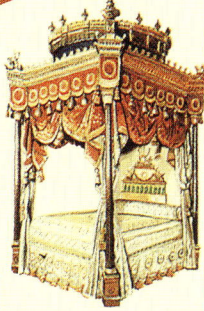

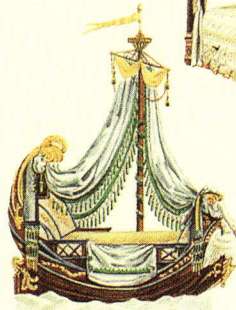

Bed shaped like a swan, French, mid 19th century

Western beds are made up of a base with a mattress on top.

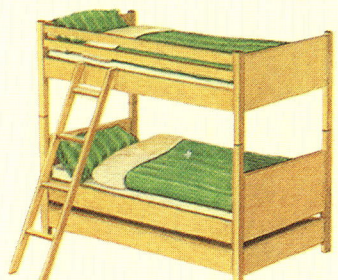

Have you slept in a bunk-bed like this one?

Who do you look like?

When a baby is born, everyone tries to see who it looks like! We all inherit features from our parents: our skin shade, the colour of our eyes and hair, the shape of our face, our voice, and even our talents and shortcomings too... It's called heredity. These special characteristics that we recognize are passed on through our genes. Are you like your father or your mother, your uncle or your aunt?

Look at the colour of other peoples' eyes.

Brown eyes are far more common world-wide than blue eyes. See how some eyes have several different shades of colour.

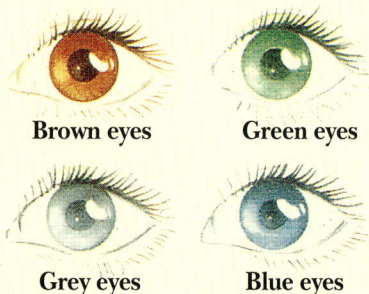

Brown eyes   **Green eyes**

Grey eyes   **Blue eyes**

Look at the members of your family: in what way do they look alike, how are they different? Don't forget that features come through your father and your mother, who have inherited genes from their own parents, so your nose may be like your granny's! You even inherited the character of your tongue: some can roll their tongue, others can't.

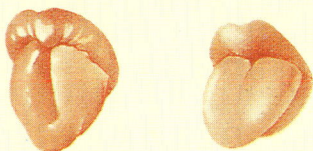

Can you?

Can you believe your eyes?

Sometimes our brain is deceived by what our eyes have seen. Optical illusions give us false information, so that our brain cannot interpret the image correctly.

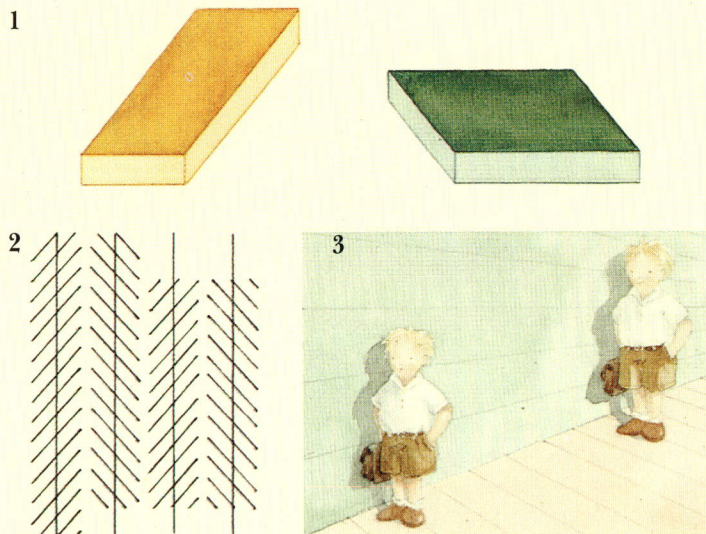

1

2   3

1. Do these two shapes look the same to you?
Trace over one, then lay the tracing over the other shape. Does it fit?

2. Are the vertical lines parallel?
Yes, they are.

3. Which of these figures is taller?
Use a ruler to check. Were you surprised by the answer?

4. Are the smaller squares below all the same size?
Yes, they are.

5. Stare at these black squares for a moment.
You will see grey dots appear where the lines intersect. If you move the paper away a little, the spots will be even more noticeable.

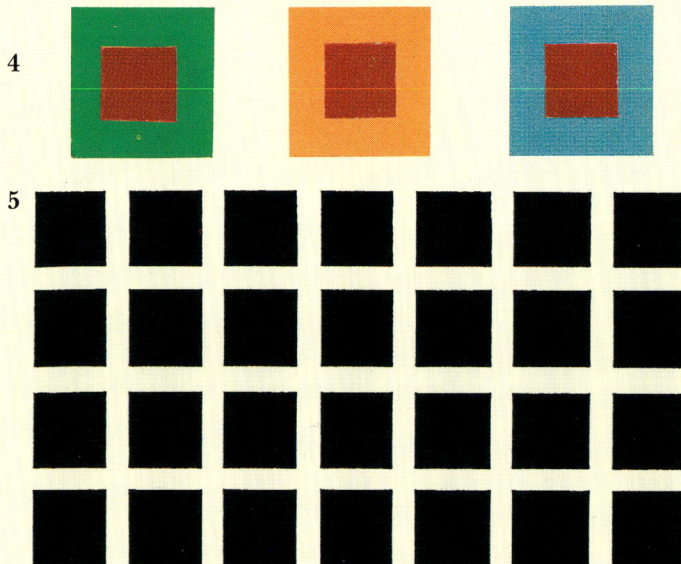

4

5

Fingerprints

Everybody's finger-prints are different.

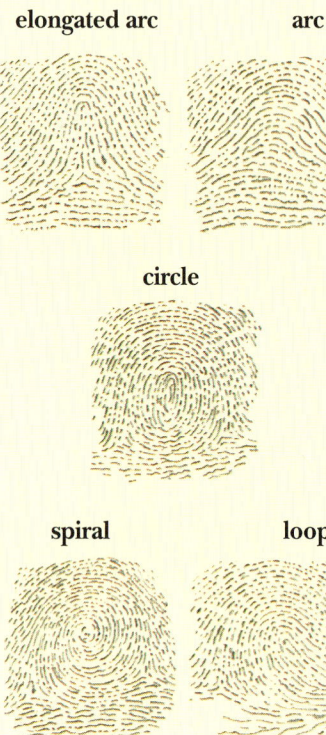

elongated arc   **arc**

circle

spiral   **loop**

To take a fingerprint, rub a piece of paper all over with a soft pencil until it's nice and black. Press your finger onto the paper. Put a piece of sticky tape over your blackened fingertip, peel back the tape and press it onto some white paper. Now see what kind of fingerprint you've got.

Even identical twins can often have different fingerprints.

What shape are the lobes of your ear?

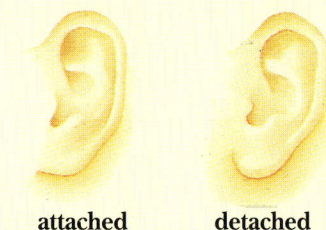

attached   **detached**

Some people can't tell the difference between red and green, or more rarely, blue. They are colour-blind.

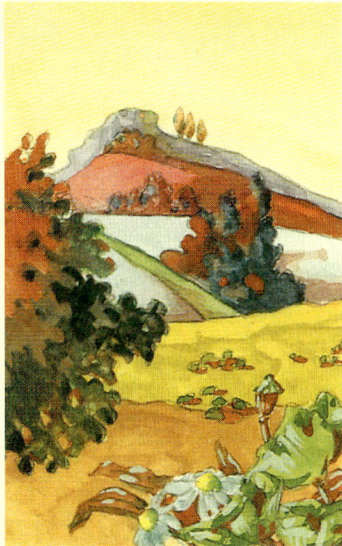

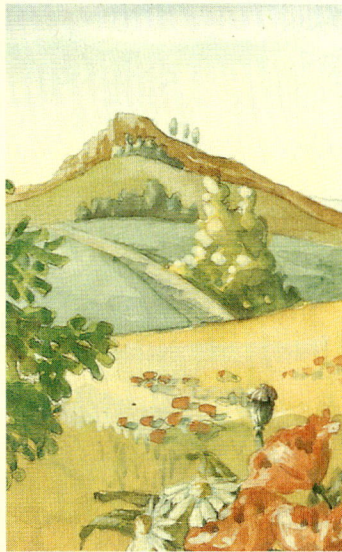

Is it possible to transplant an eye?
No, you can't replace a whole eye. But you can transplant a cornea. It's quite a simple operation nowadays, and has saved many people's sight.

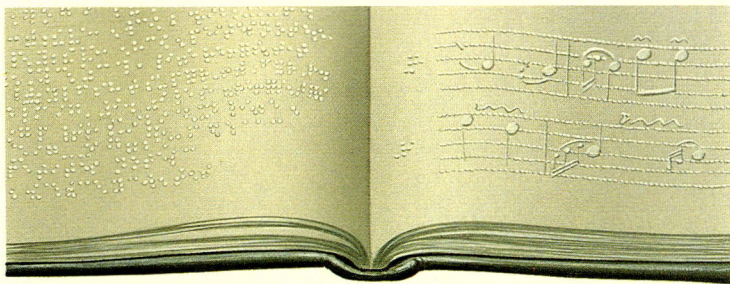

The Braille alphabet
It's impossible for people with poor sight or no sight at all to read an ordinary book. A Frenchman called Louis Braille (1809-1852), who was blind himself, invented an alphabet using a system of six raised dots, which are punched into thick paper. Blind people can learn to read books written in braille by running their fingertips over the pages. They can also read music in this way.

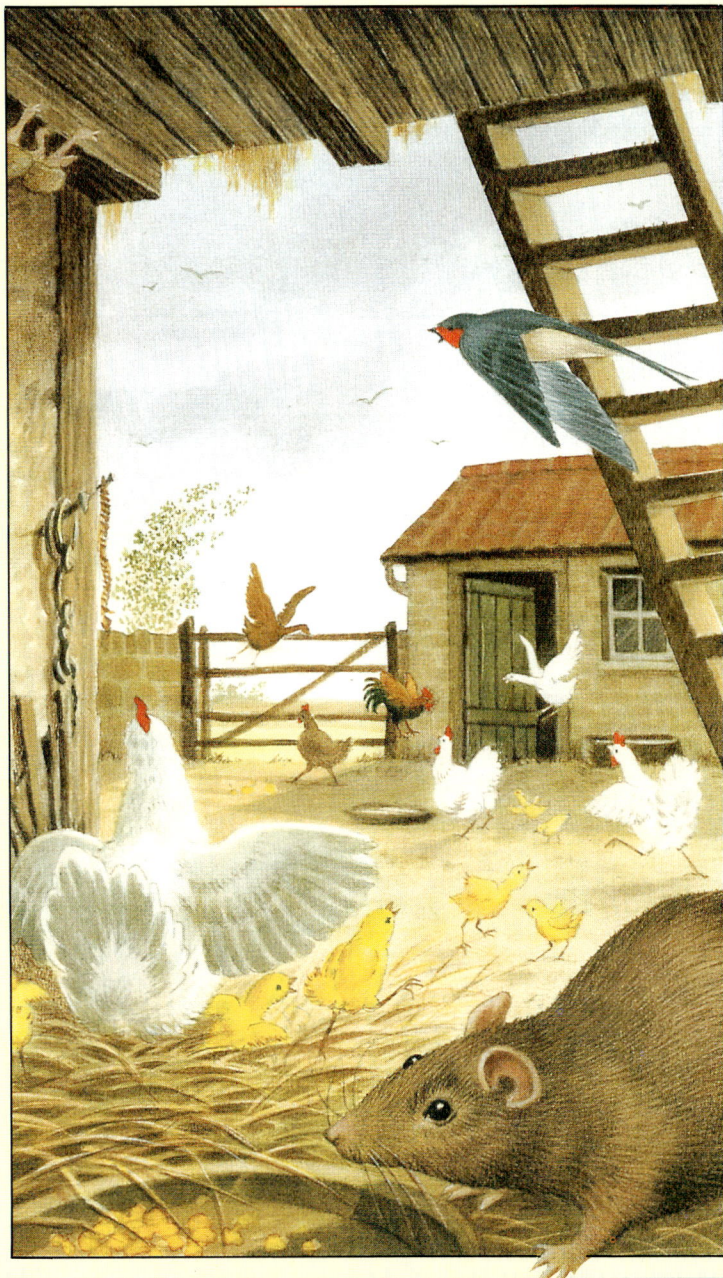

The animal with the biggest eyes
is the giant squid. Its eyes are 38 cm. in diameter!

The male silkworm
has thousands of tiny scent organs on its antennae to help it pick up smells.

Caterpillars are covered with hairs which react to sound. They can freeze at the slightest noise.

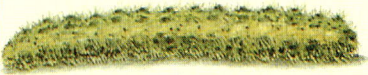

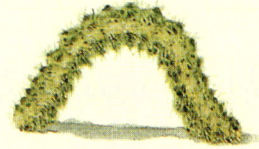

Chameleons can look in two directions at once, since their eyes swivel round independently of each other.

Tarsier

Chameleon

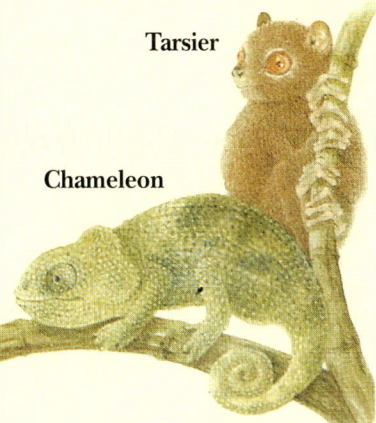

The little tarsier,
a nocturnal animal related to the lemur, has the biggest eyes in proportion to its size of any mammal.

How do doctors examine your heart?

They can listen to your heartbeat with a stethoscope*. An electrocardiogram (ECG) displays patterns of impulses, which show how healthy the heart is in more detail.

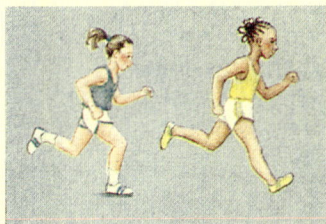

If a heart isn't working properly, or a baby is born with a heart defect, the problem may be treated with drugs or can sometimes be put right with an operation.

But occasionally the only way to save the patient's life is by heart transplant. In a long and extremely delicate operation, the diseased heart is removed and a healthy heart, taken from someone who has just met their death accidentally, is put in its place.

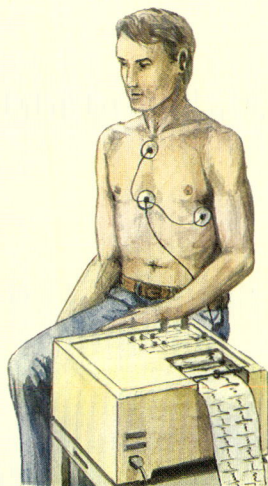

■ Did you know?

In cases of severe burns, skin tissues have been so badly damaged they are no longer able to heal on their own. Doctors perform a skin graft: a thin strip of skin is lifted from a healthy part of the patient's body, and stuck, or grafted, onto the injury, to help the wound to heal over.

There is a small number of people who do not have any pigments at all: their hair is white, their eyes are pink and their skin is pale. They are albinos. This is very uncommon in humans, but occurs more often in animals. You may have seen an albino rabbit or mouse, with pink eyes.

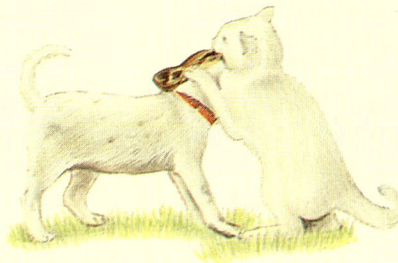

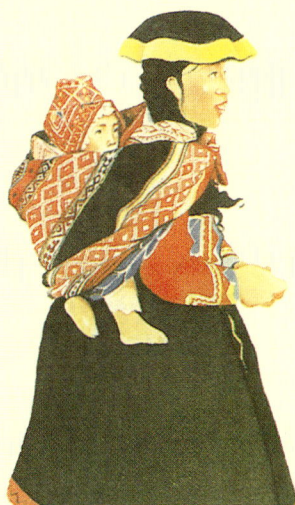

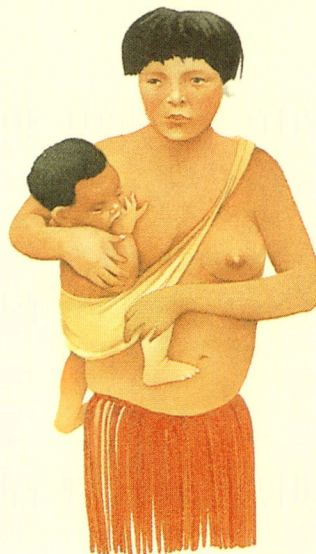

There are many variations in the colour of skin, from darkest black to freckled white.
Whatever its shade, skin is always coloured by the same pigment, called melanin.

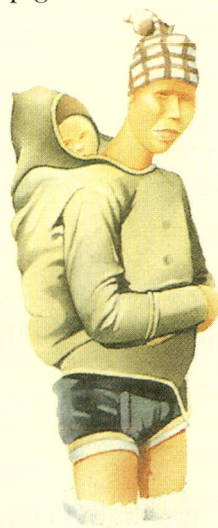

In a pale skin, melanin is concentrated in one small space in each skin cell. In a dark skin, melanin spreads out, darkening the whole cell. So the colour of a person's skin does not depend on the amount of melanin, but on how widely it is distributed.

A new, useful germ has just been discovered!

It's a germ which eats cars! Industrialists in the old East Germany were not very concerned about pollution and had produced three million plastic cars, all giving off very dirty exhaust gases. Something had to be done. Two German biologists have discovered a bacteria which devours bodywork: it takes twenty days to get rid of 650 kilos of plastic! So you see, some germs really can be useful!

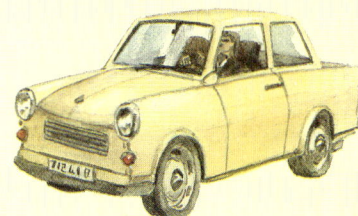

Rhythms of the heart

A baby's heartbeat is very fast at birth: 140 times per minute. An adult's resting heartbeat is about 75 times a minute. The rhythm speeds up when you exercise. It isn't good for your heart to beat either too fast or too slowly. It beats faster when you have a temperature. If you're very frightened, your heart can stop for a split second, then start again: it has literally 'missed a beat'.

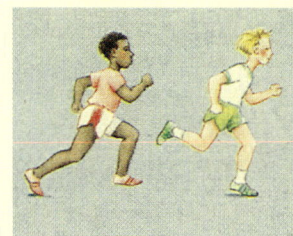

Human ears can't pick up every sound. Some of the noises you hear are more high-pitched than others. The higher the sound, the more soundwave vibrations it gives out each second. The soundwaves are measured in units called Hertz, or Hz for short.

Sounds below 20 Hz are too low for us to hear, and they are known as infra-sounds. The human voice has a range of between 200 and 4,000 Hz. Like a cat, a new-born baby can hear sounds of up to 30,000 Hz. A child can hear up to 20,000 Hz, an adult of 30 up to 16,000 Hz, a fifty-year-old man up to 8,000 Hz and an old person of eighty, just 4,000 Hz. We cannot hear any sound above 20,000 Hz: these are called ultrasounds.

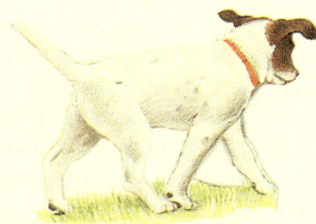

Dogs can hear sounds up to 40,000 Hz. But the ultrasound champions are dolphins and bats: they can hear up to 150,000 Hz!

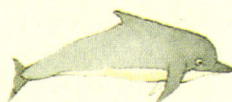

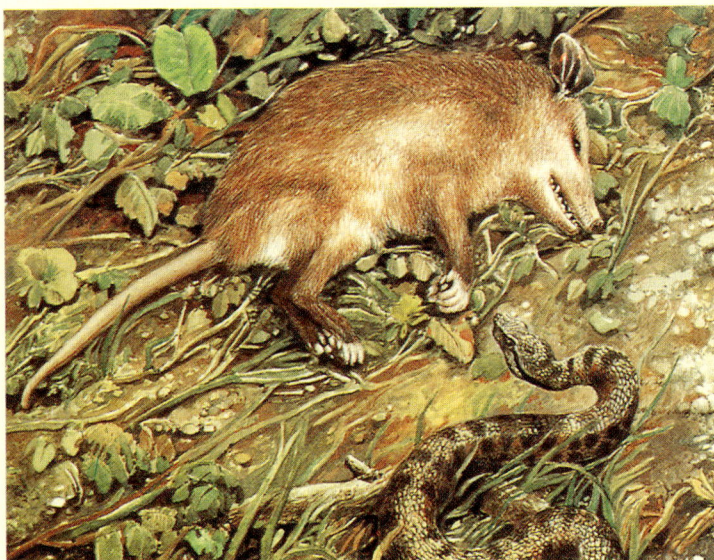

Opossums fall into a kind of trance, hypnotized by the swaying of a snake.

A different kind of sleep

Hypnosis is a sort of sleep brought about by a special use of words and gestures or sounds. People who are hypnotized look as though they are asleep, but they can still hear and obey orders. Some animals have the power to hypnotize. Their prey is so fascinated by their movements that it is unable to move, until suddenly the killer springs. A mongoose can even hypnotize and kill a snake in this way.

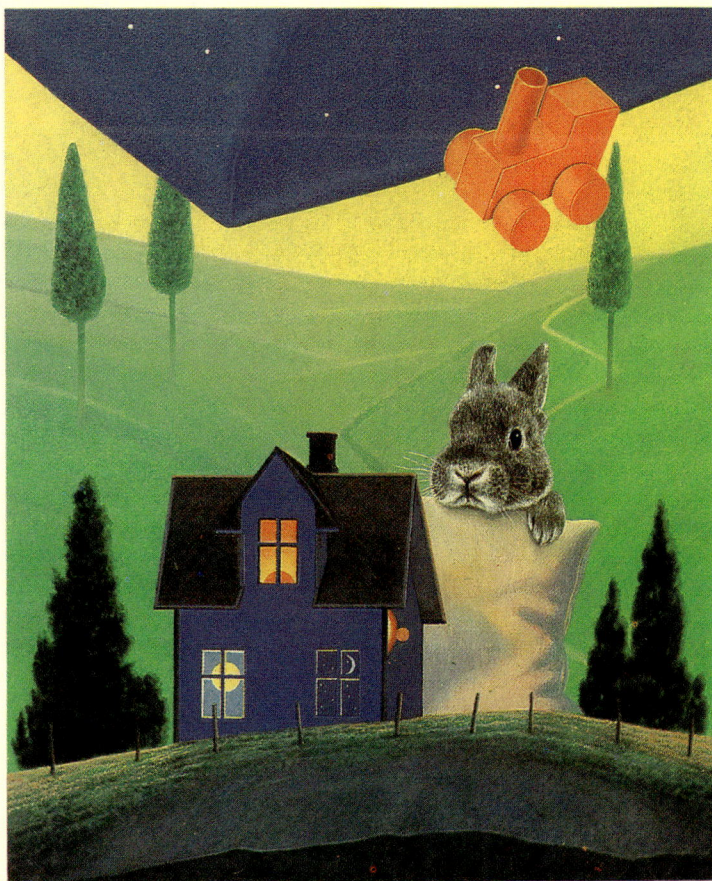

Deaf people often use a sign language to communicate. Sign language is made up of hand movements, which can be made very rapidly and understood in an instant. Deaf people also become very good at lip-reading. Highly sophisticated hearing aids can help some people pick up certain sounds.

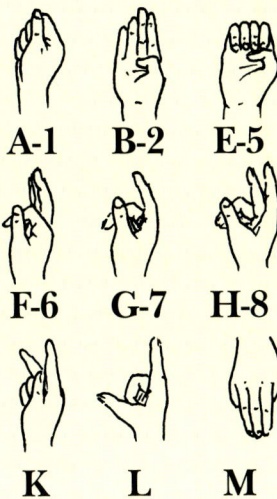

A-1   B-2   E-5

F-6   G-7   H-8

K   L   M

Some drugs come from plants, others are chemically produced. All drugs act on neurones, the nerve cells which link every different part of the body to the brain. Gradually, drugs destroy a person's neurones, even if they are not aware of the damage being done. But once a neurone is destroyed, it is gone for good. Neurones can never be replaced!

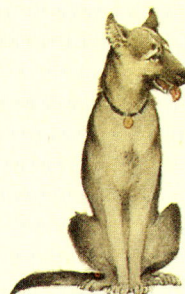

There's only one correct answer to each question. See if you can get the answer right! Check your answers with the solutions at the bottom of page 71.

1. While a baby is in its mother's tummy, the umbilical cord helps it...
   a) not to float away
   b) to feed
   c) to develop its muscles

2. Which of these organs only starts to work once a baby is born?
   a) the heart
   b) the brain
   c) the lungs

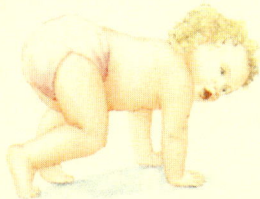

3. A baby begins to hear...
   a) when it's in its mother's tummy
   b) when it's born
   c) a few days after birth

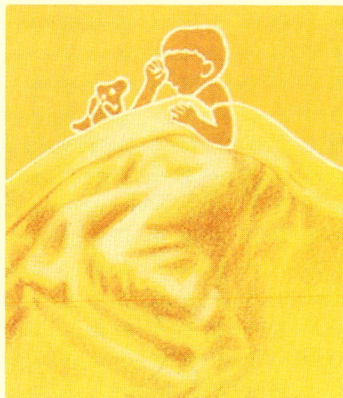

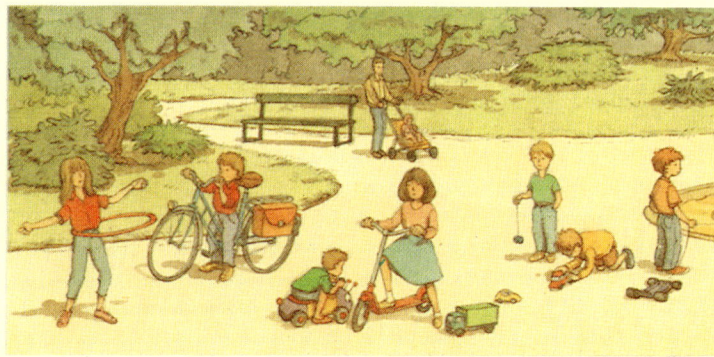

4. How many genes does a human being have?
   a) about 50,000
   b) more than 10 million
   c) 23 pairs

5. As your heart pumps, oxygenated blood and stale blood...
   a) sometimes mix
   b) never mix
   c) are mixing all the time

6. Your sense of balance is found in...
   a) your brain
   b) your ears
   c) your legs

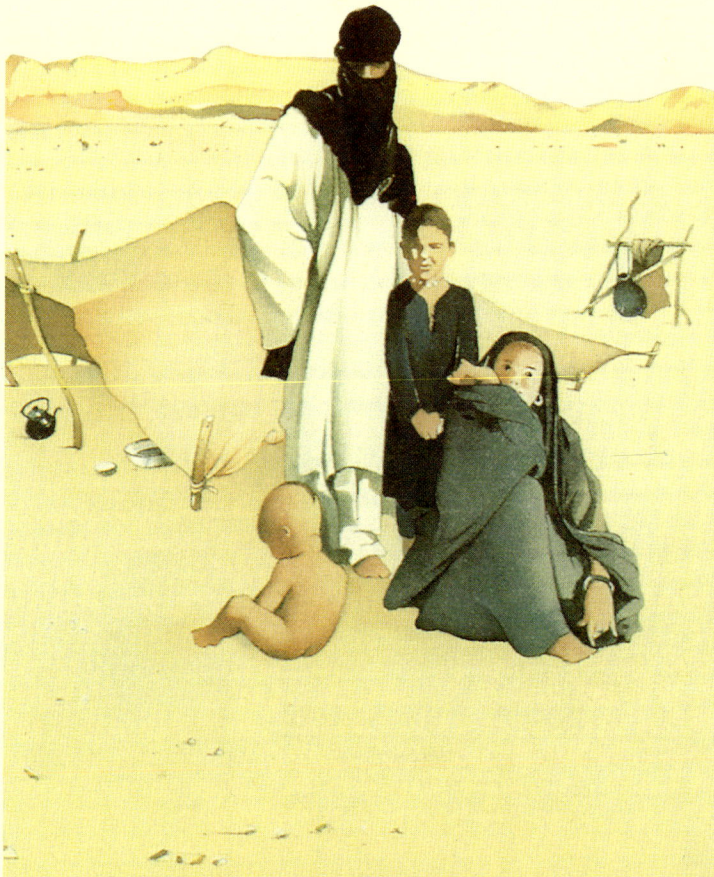

7. Which organ in your body needs germs to help it work properly?
   a) the brain
   b) the heart
   c) the intestine

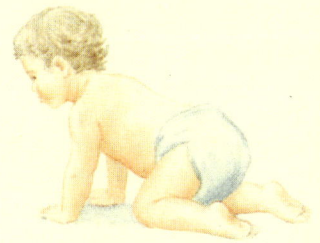

8. The word 'virus' is a Latin word, meaning:
   a) poison
   b) vein
   c) tiny

9. Which of these tools is difficult for someone who is left-handed?
   a) a knife
   b) a saw
   c) a pair of scissors

10. The size of the pupil in the centre of the eye varies depending on...
   a) your age
   b) what you are thinking about
   c) the amount of light

11. Because we have two eyes, we are able to see things...
   a) in detail
   b) from both sides at once
   c) in three dimensions

12. If you can see close-up things clearly, but not distant things, you are:
   a) short-sighted
   b) long-sighted
   c) colour-blind

True or false?

1. Antibodies are a type of virus.

2. Not eating breakfast in the morning is a good way to slim.

3. All vitamins can be found in the body.

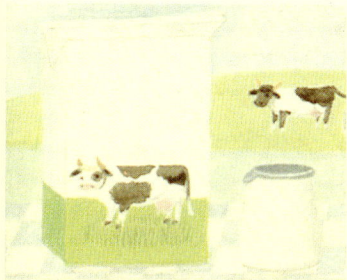

4. Genes are so tiny that you cannot see them, even with a microscope.

5. The study of similarities between parents and their children is called genetic science.

6. Laid end to end, all the blood vessels in your body would measure 150,000 km.

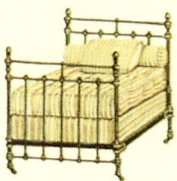

7. Antibiotics kill bacteria and viruses.

8. The sex of a baby is decided the moment the egg is fertilized.

9. The two sides of your heart are completely separate from each other.

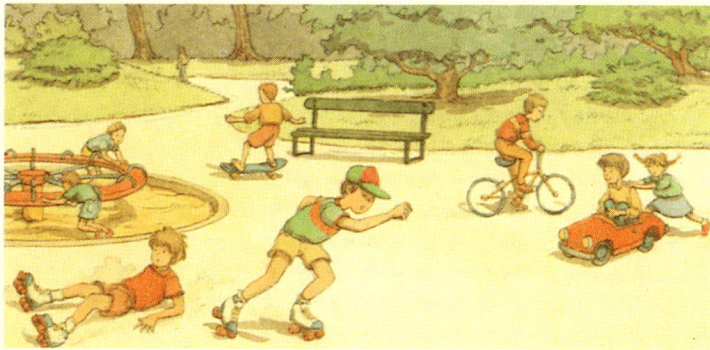

10. Veins leave your heart and arteries return to it.

11. Blood cells are made in your bone marrow.

12. When you are asleep, your brain is resting too.

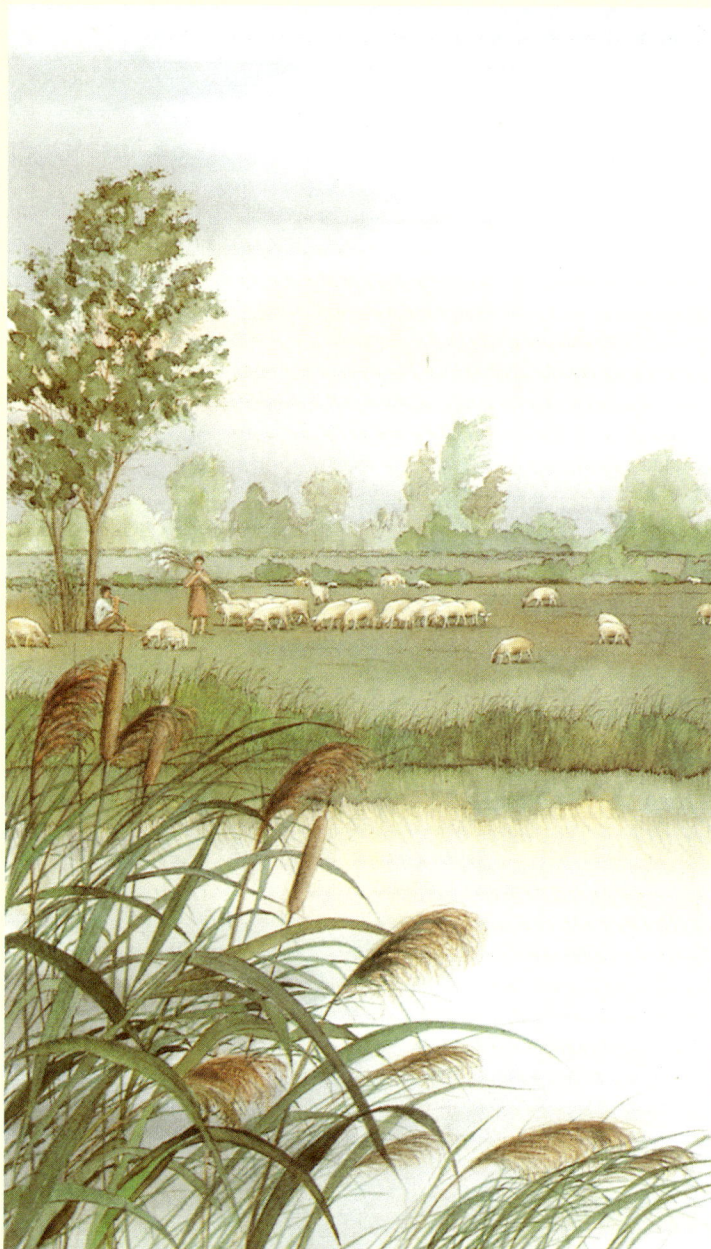

Do you know the answers to these questions?

1. What did the painter Leonardo da Vinci, the musician Ludwig van Beethoven, and the comic actor Charlie Chaplin have in common?
They were all left-handed.

2. If you are 'ambidextrous', what can you do?
Use both your right and left hands equally well.

3. How tall are African pygmies?
They are the smallest race of people in the world. None of them is taller than 1.45 m.

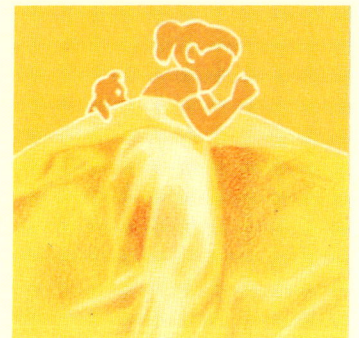

Answers:

Quiz
1.b - 2.c - 3.a - 4.a - 5.b - 6.b - 7.c - 8.a - 9.c - 10.c - 11.c - 12.a

True or false
1. False. Antibodies are substances made by the body to help fight off disease.
2. False. Your body needs energy in the morning, as it has had no fuel for 12 hours.
3. False. Vitamins are found in food.
4. True.
5. True.
6. True. Nearly four times round the Earth.
7. False. Only bacteria.
8. True.
9. True.
10. False. It's the opposite.
11. True.
12. False. Your brain is very active, sorting out the events of the day, and dreaming.

Allergy: a reaction, like a running nose, a rash or wheezing, suffered by people sensitive to certain substances, foods or even medicines. At least one person in ten has an allergy occasionally.

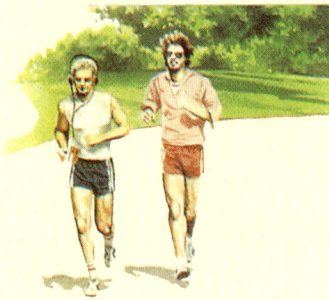

Anaesthetic: a substance which takes away the patient's sensitivity to pain. A general anaesthetic sends you to sleep before an operation. An anaesthetist is the doctor in charge of keeping you in this state of artificial sleep. A local anaesthetic simply numbs a small area for a short time, so that a wound can be stitched up, for instance. The dentist gives you a local anaesthetic when he has to drill a tooth.

Antibiotics: drugs which can kill bacteria, by preventing them growing or reproducing. They do not kill viruses, and so cannot cure virus diseases such as colds or 'flu. Penicillin is still the most commonly used antibiotic.

Auditory: connected with hearing.

Booster: a second dose of a vaccine, given at a later date to increase the amount of antibodies and give extra protection. Children in the U.K. have a pre-school booster of the vaccines they were given as babies, (except whooping-cough), at the age of about four and a half.

Cartilage: soft, elastic white tissue which covers the ends of bones at the joints. It's also found in your nose and ear lobes.

Cetacean: member of the family of mammals containing whales and dolphins.

Cholesterol: a fatty substance found in foods like egg yolk and shellfish. A high level of cholesterol in the blood can lead to hardening of the arteries and heart disease, particularly in men.

Constipation: if your intestines cannot get rid of undigested food, because of lack of fibre (roughage) or water in your diet, this solid waste matter becomes hard and dry. You are constipated. It's difficult to go to the toilet and you begin to have a tummy ache.

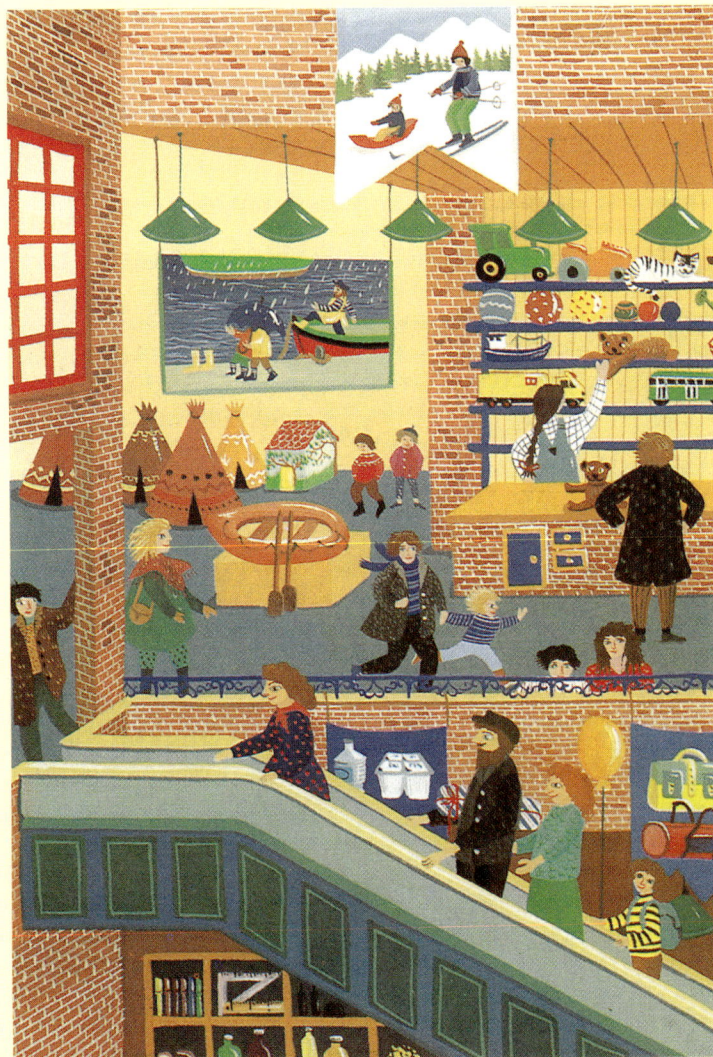

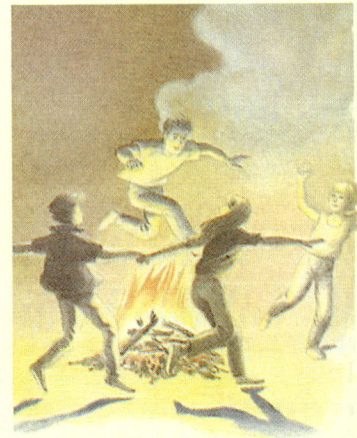

to Diagnose: to discover what disease someone has from looking at their symptoms and sometimes carrying out tests. A doctor must make an accurate diagnosis in order to treat a patient successfully.

Fertilization: the moment when the sperm penetrates the ovum, and the first cell of a new baby is made. This is known as the moment of conception.

Gastro-enteritis: inflammation of the stomach and intestines, often caused by a virus. It usually leads to stomach-aches, vomiting and diarrhoea. Vital body fluids are quickly lost and have to be replaced.

Gene: chromosomes are made up of genes. Each person has between 50,000 and 100,000 of them. Chromosomes are rather like the memory of a computer. The genes they carry hold the plans for the make-up of our entire body, including all the characteristics special to us, in a very complicated chemical called DNA.

Health Visitor: a special nurse who works in the community, not in hospital, giving advice to parents on the health of babies and children. She also advises elderly people how to keep well.

Immunity: if you are immune to an illness, your body has built up a stock of antibodies against it and you will not fall ill. You can become immune by having vaccinations or by just coming into contact with a disease.

Membrane: a thin skin, covering organs such as the heart and lungs, and lining the nose, mouth and intestine. Many lining membranes produce mucus, a moistening, lubricating and protective fluid, and they are then known as mucous membranes.

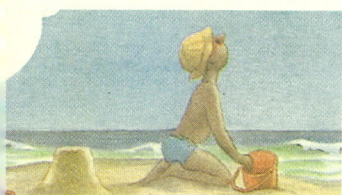

Nucleus: the central part of a cell, containing the chromosomes.

Oxygen: we could not live without oxygen, a colourless, odourless gas found in the air we breathe.

Parasite: an animal (or plant) that lives in or on another living thing, taking its food from it.

Penis: one of the male sex organs, also used for passing urine out of the body.

Periods: when a girl reaches puberty, she produces a mature ovum every 28 days or so. The uterus grows a thick lining just in case the egg is fertilized and becomes an embryo. If this doesn't happen, the lining is shed, along with some blood, down through the vagina. This bleeding is known as a period, or menstruation, and normally lasts about 4 or 5 days in each month.

Pigment: the substance that gives your skin, hair and eyes their colour.

Pituitary gland: gland at the base of the brain which produces and releases several hormones. These include growth hormones and those which stimulate a man's testes to produce sperm, and the ovaries in a woman to develop egg cells.

Plaque: a harmful film which forms on the teeth. It can be controlled by careful brushing and flossing and regular visits to the dentist.

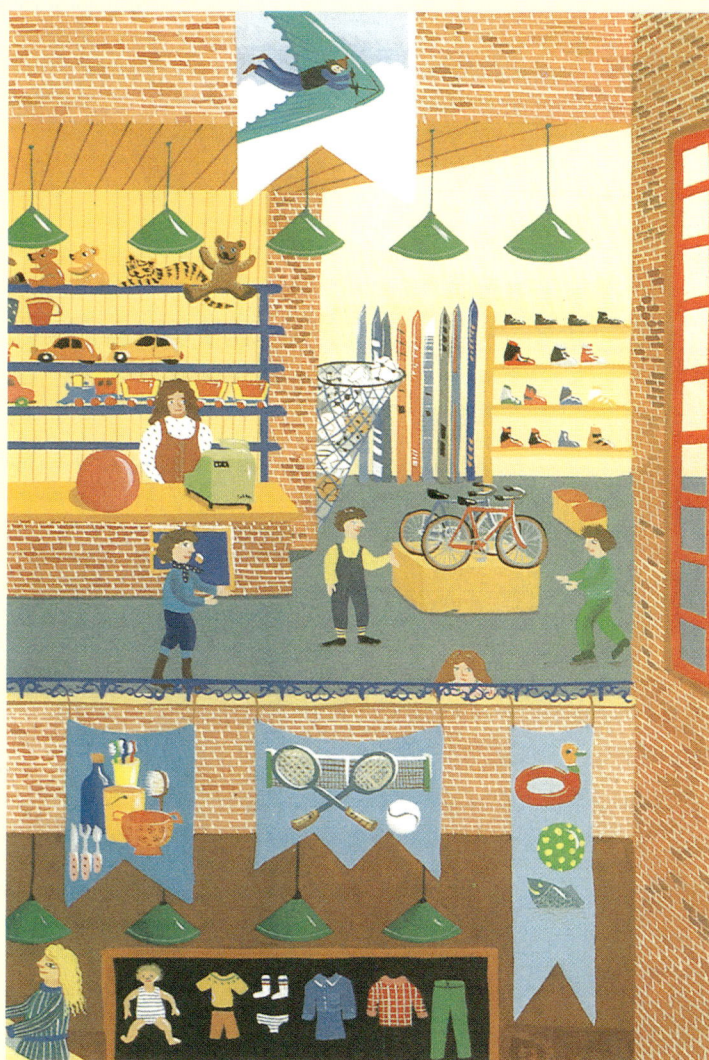

Saliva: fluid produced by glands in the mouth. Saliva moistens food so that it can be swallowed easily.

Stethoscope: instrument used by a doctor to hear what is going on inside the body.

Tissues: groups of similar cells which are bound together to form various parts of the body; for instance muscle tissue, or nerve tissue.

Vaccination: a way of protecting ourselves from certain illnesses, by injecting a small dose of the weakened or dead bacteria or virus. This stimulates the body's natural defence system to produce antibodies against the disease.

Vagina: the passageway from the uterus to the outside of a girl's body. In an adult woman it is about 10-12 cm long. It is made of muscle lined with membrane. During childbirth the vagina stretches as the baby passes through.

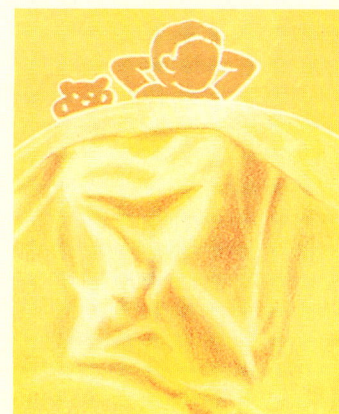

■ Accidents and Emergencies

Accidents and emergencies happen very quickly and without warning. It might be that the person who needs your help can't even talk to you. What can you do to help?

When you go to help someone you must make sure that you are in no danger yourself. If you think there is any risk of your being injured, tell the person who is hurt to stay still while you get an adult to help you.

When someone is hurt there is a set of rules that you should follow. And remember: never give an injured person anything to eat, drink or smoke.

Is the person awake and able to talk to you? If they are not awake, tilt their head back and lift the chin up. Keep doing this and put your ear down by their mouth and nose. Listen for their breathing and watch to see if their chest rises and falls. Listen and watch while you count to five. If the person is breathing, turn him onto his side and keep his head tilted back. If he is not breathing, do not waste any time – go and get help; dial 999 and ask for an ambulance.

If you have been on a First Aid course, you might know how to give mouth to mouth resuscitation.

Someone who is hurt is suffering from shock and needs extra warmth – cover them with warm clothing or a blanket.

Fainting
If someone gets very hot or has a bad shock, they may faint. Lift their legs as high as you can. If they don't wake up after 2 or 3 minutes, follow the instructions above.

Cuts
If someone is badly cut, it's important to stop the bleeding. All you need to do is apply direct pressure to the wound: do this with your hand by pushing onto the wound. At the same time, try and keep the affected limb up above the person's body. If you have a clean handkerchief or similar, make a pad, put that on the wound and press on it.

Broken bones
If someone has been knocked down, has fallen heavily or has been in an accident, they may have broken a bone. The affected limb will be painful and may be an unusual shape. Tell the person not to move. Hold the injured limb above and below the suspected break, to support it and keep it still.

Burns and scalds
If someone burns or scalds themselves, you must cool the affected area by putting it in cold water until the pain has gone. If a person's clothes catch fire, quickly wrap them in a blanket. When the flames have gone out, put cold water on the burns.

Choking
If a person gets something stuck in their windpipe, they will choke. Move the person so that their head is lower than their waist, then tap them sharply between the shoulder-blades, 4 or 5 times.

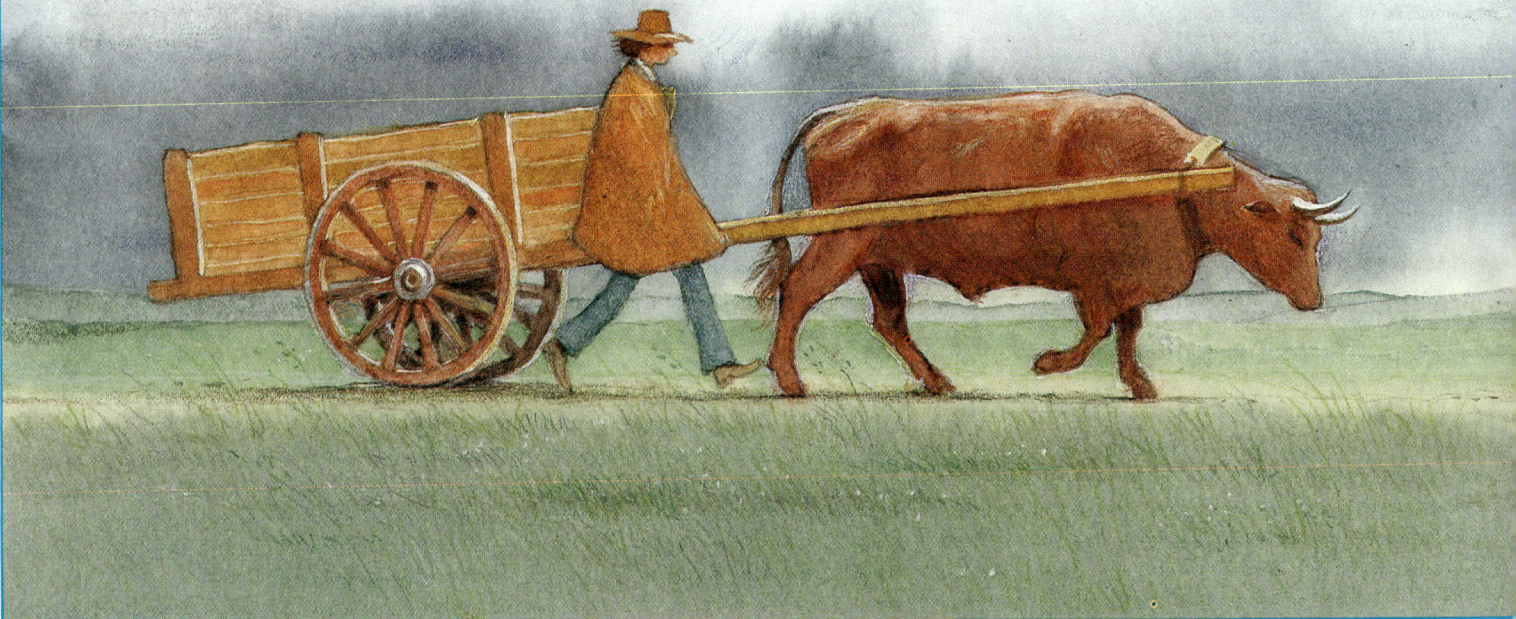

Dialling 999

The telephone call is free.
**Ask for an ambulance.
Answer all the questions clearly and give
the following information:**

Full address or place of the accident or emergency –
be as clear and precise as you can.

Some idea of the type of accident

Some idea of the number of casualties (that is people
who are hurt)

If it's a road accident and you are on a motorway,
the emergency telephones are situated every mile
and the 100 metre marker posts will tell you where
the nearest phone is. If there is no adult who can go,
climb up the bank and walk to the phone to call
the ambulance. Don't forget to explain that you are
on your own without adult help.

Checklist for what to do in an emergency

If the person is not awake...put them on their side,
with their head tilted back.

If the person is bleeding...press on the wound
and raise the cut part of the body.

If the person might have broken a bone...keep it
as still as you can.

If the person has a burn or scald...put cold water on it.

Cover the person with a blanket.

Go and get help.

■ First Aid Training

First Aid training teaches you how to help someone
who is injured.
The British Red Cross and St. John Ambulance run
First Aid courses. Ask at your school or your local library
for details of courses, or contact:

British Red Cross
National Headquarters
9 Grosvenor Crescent
London SW1X 7EJ

St. John Ambulance
National Headquarters
1 Grosvenor Crescent
London SW1X 7EF

St. Andrew's Ambulance Association
St. Andrew's House
Milton Street
Glasgow G4 0RH

The Order of Malta
32 Drumnagreagh Road
Cairncastle
Larne BT40 2RP

*These pages have been written
with the help of Anthony Kemp, SRN IFNA,
Senior Training Officer in First Aid
at the British Red Cross. His advice
is gratefully acknowledged.*

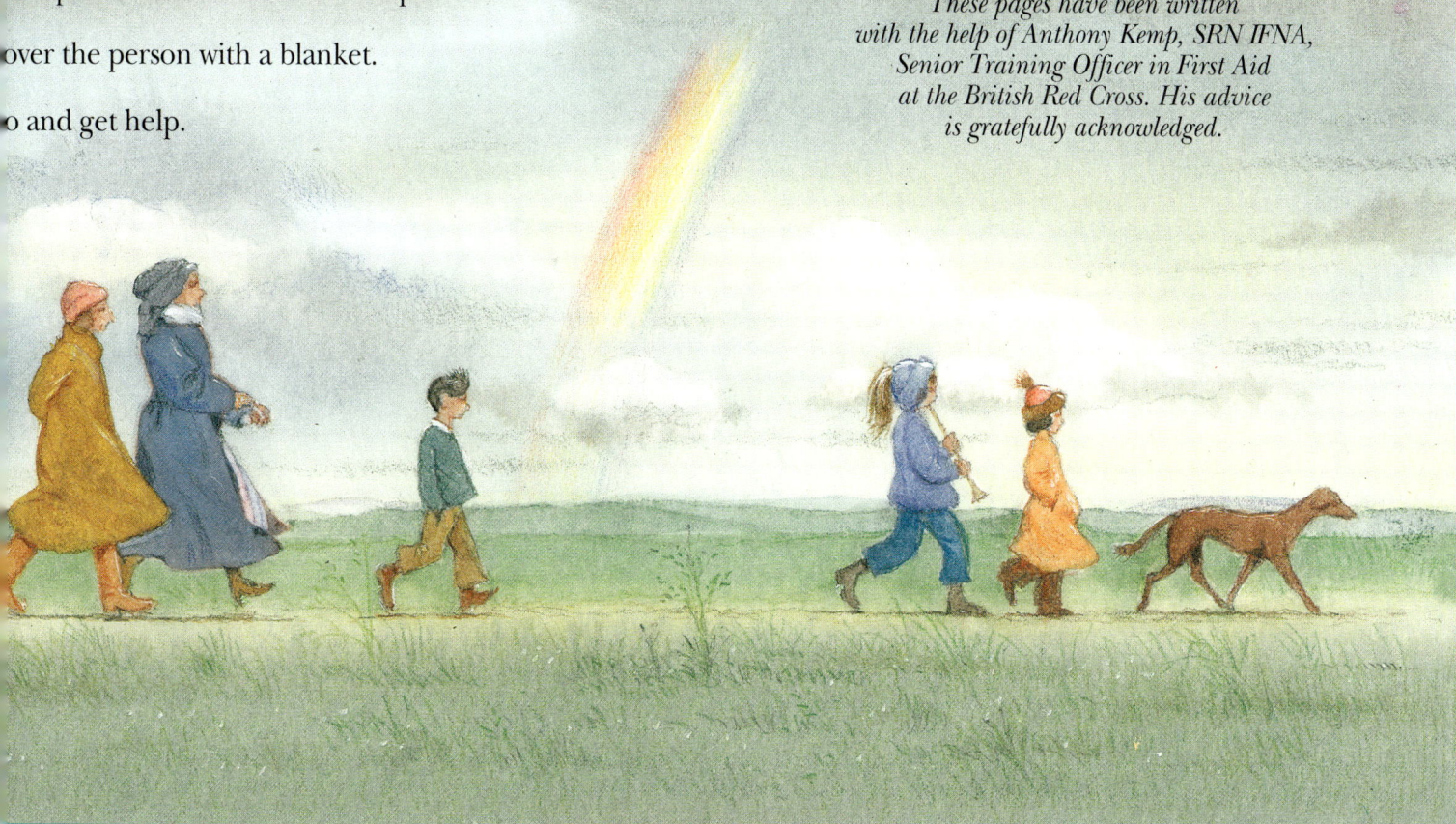

INDEX

Hospital, If you are seriously ill or you need an operation...you will be looked after in hospital, 56-57; *see also* 12, 25, 28
Hygiene, 58
Hypnosis, 69

I **Illness,** Some germs are friendly, others are harmful, 53, The unending battle against disease, 55; *see also* 54
Immunity, 53, 73
Incubator, 11
Indigestion, 17
Infection, 28, 29, 52, 53
Intestine, 16, 17, 34, 52

J Jawbone, 19
Joint, 33

K **Kidney,** Your kidneys help to get rid of your body's waste, 30; *see also* 17

L Labour, 12
Ligament, 33
Liver, 16, 17
Lungs, You have been breathing since the moment you were born, 24, Your lungs fill up with air, 24; *see also* 11, 16, 28
Lymphatic system, 29, 37, 52, 53

M Malnutrition, 59
Mammal, 7
Melanin, 37, 68
Membrane, 73
Muscles, Walking...Running...Jumping, 34, Muscles work hard to allow us to move about, 35; *see also* 39, 40

N Neurone, 38, 39, 40, 50, 69
Nipple, 12
Nutrients, 16, 17

O Oesophagus, 16
Operation, 56
Ophthalmologist, 42
Optic nerve, 42
Orbit, 42
Ovary, 30, 31
Ovum, 8
Oxygen, 24, 73

P Paediatric ward, 57
Pain, 47
Parasite, 52, 73
Pasteur, Louis Pasteur: the pioneer of vaccination, 54
Pasteurization, 54
Penis, 8, 30, 73
Periods, 31, 73
Personal hygiene, 58
Personality, 15
Pituitary gland, 15, 73
Placenta, 10, 12, 64
Plaque, 21, 73
Plasma, 28
Platelet, 28, 29
Pneumonia, 25
Pregnancy, Nine months...to form a new person, 10-11, The magical moment of birth, 12; *see also* 9
Premature baby, 11
Protein, 22
Puberty, 15, 31
Pulmonary artery, 27
Pulse, 27
Pupil, 42, 70

R Rabies, 54
Reproductive system, Genital organs to make babies when you are grown-up, 31

Respiratory system, You have been breathing since the moment you were born, 24, Your lungs fill up with air, 24; *see also* 11, 16
Retina, 42
Ribcage, 32

S Saliva, 16, 21, 73
Scrotum, 30
Sea-sickness, 44
Sebum, 37
Semi-circular canals, 44
Senses, We experience the world with our five senses, 40
It's up to us to use and develop our senses, 41
Sight, The eye is a very delicate organ, 42, If your vision isn't perfect glasses can help you to see better, 43
Sign language, 69
Sixth sense, 41
Skeleton, Your skeleton has 208 bones holding you upright, 32, It's a framework that's very much alive! 33
Skin, From your head to your toes, your body is wrapped in skin, 36, It's important to look after your skin, 37, The sense of touch is located in the skin, 47; *see also* 52
Smoking, 25, 27
Sleep, At the end of every day...our body and mind need sleep, 47-48, Each night, you go through several stages of sleep, 50, Your brain can be busy while you're asleep, 51; *see also* 58, 59
Smell, Your nose can pick up several thousand different smells, 45-46; *see also* 47
Sperm, 8, 9, 30, 31
Spine, 6, 38
Spots, 31
Stethoscope, 26, 68, 73
Stomach, 16, 17, 34
Sugar, 21, 22, 23
Swelling, 37
Synovial fluid, 33

T **Taste,** How do we taste things? We use our tongues, 46
Teeth, Your teeth are on show when you smile! 18, Teeth are little bones planted in your gums, 19, Milk teeth and permanent teeth, 20, Take good care of your teeth! 21,
Tendon, 34
Testicle, 30, 31
Tetanus, 53
Tissue, 14, 37, 73
Tongue, 18, 46, 66
Touch, The sense of touch is located in the skin, 47
Tuberculosis, 53
Tumour, 53
Twins, 9, 66
Tympanum, 44

U Ultrasound, 69
Umbilical cord, 10, 13, 70
Urine, 17, 30, 56
Uterus, 30
Uvula, 18

V **Vaccination,** Louis Pasteur: the pioneer of vaccination, 54; *see also* 53, 55, 59, 73
Vagina, 8, 12, 30, 73
Valve, 27
Vertebrae, 38
Virus, The unending battle against disease, 55; *see also* 17, 52, 53, 70
Vitamins, What good does good food do? 23; *see also* 17, 19, 22, 61
Vocal cords, 24

W Water, 22, 23
Wet-nurse, 64
Worms, 17

X X-ray, 20, 33, 56, 57

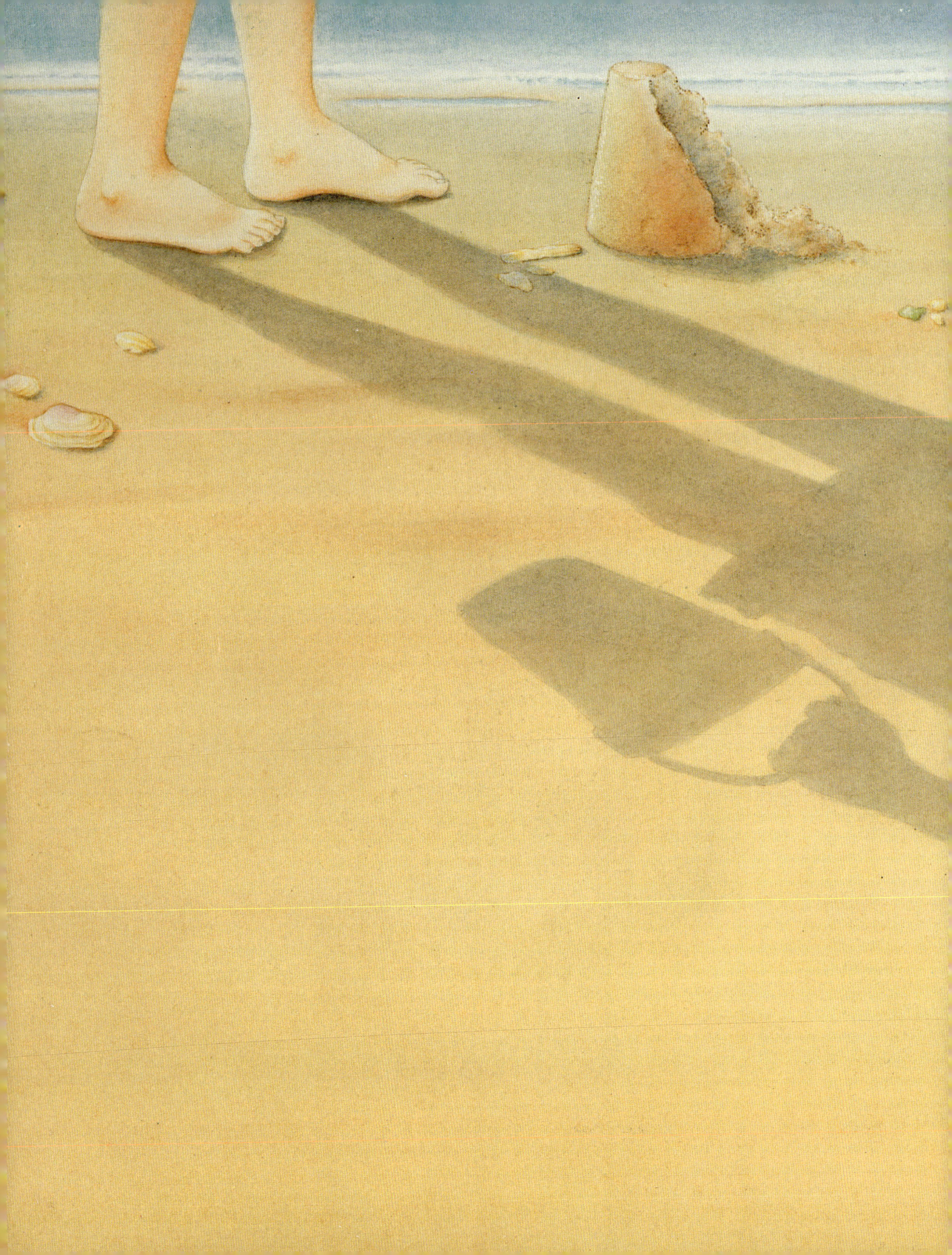